The CYCLIST'S F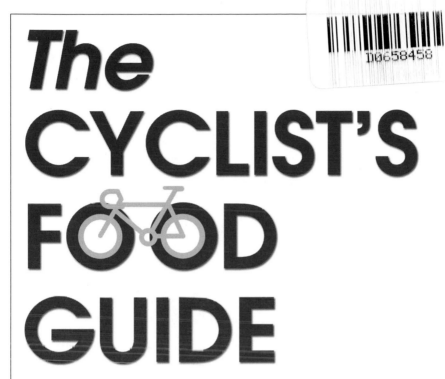D GUIDE

FUELING FOR THE DISTANCE

Nancy Clark, MS, RD
Jenny Hegmann, MS, RD

Foreword by Michael McCoy
Adventure Cycling Association

Sports Nutrition Publishers
West Newton, MA

Clark, Nancy 1951- Hegmann, Jenny 1965 -
    The Cyclist's Food Guide: Fueling for the Distance
    p. cm
    Includes bibliographical references and index.
    LCCN 2004107717
    ISBN 0-9718911-1-7

    1. Sports—Nutrition 2. Bicycle riding
    I. Title

Complete Cataloging-in-Publication Data available on request

Book design by Patricia Robinson, Waban, MA patrobinsondesign@comcast.net

Cover photo: Adventure Cycling Association photo by Aaron Teasdale

Published in West Newton, MA, by Sports Nutrition Publishers
60 Lindbergh Avenue Suite 2A, West Newton MA 02465
617-795-0823   sportsnutrition@rcn.com

This book is available at special discounts for bulk purchase. Special editions or book excerpts can also be created to specification. For details, contact the sales manager at Sports Nutrition Publishers.

Printed in the United States of America 10 9 8 7 6 5 4 3 2 1

The information contained in this book is not intended to serve as a substitute for professional medical advice. The authors and publisher specifically disclaim any and all liability arising directly or indirectly from the use of any information contained in this book. A health care professional should be consulted regarding your specific medical and nutritional concerns.

♻ Printed on recycled paper using soy-based ink.

*We dedicate this book to the cyclists who give
of their time and energy to raise money for important
causes and help make the world a better place.
We want to help these everyday champions to eat
effectively, so they can enjoy high energy,
good health, and miles of enjoyable cycling.*

CONTENTS

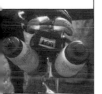
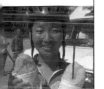
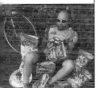

ACKNOWLEDGMENTS

F IRST OF ALL, WE OFFER ABUNDANT THANKS TO ADVENTURE CYCLING ASSOCIATION for their generosity in providing many of the photographs in this book and for their whole-hearted support for this project. Particular thanks goes to Greg Siple and Mike McCoy.

Many thanks also go to John Hughes, the managing director of UltraMarathon Cycling Association for providing photographs of ultra cycling events as well as enthusiastic interest in our project.

We appreciate the help from scores of cyclists all over the world—the randonneurs, cyclo-tourists, mountain bikers, racers, and recreational riders—who eagerly shared their personal food stories and nutrition tips.

We send our personal thanks to—
- Our loving families for their enthusiastic and supportive cheers.
- Paul, Jenny's chief support-crew, for so patiently waiting for her at the finish line of book completion.
- Pat Robinson, graphic artist, for creating a nice book from our words.
- John McGrath, Nancy's husband and business partner, for his publishing skills, wisdom, and never-ending support.
- Mark McMaster for providing racing photographs.
- The many cyclists who have helped us understand their nutrition concerns—the clients, coaches, and cycling friends both near and far—especially Lon Haldeman, Adam Hodges Myerson of Cycle-Smart, Inc., Northampton, Mass., Bruce Ingle, Skip and Danielle Komisar, Ed Kross, Rich Lesnik, MaryAnn Martinez, Mark McMaster, the Northeast Bicycle Club, and Jessica Truslow. Their experiences help us to better help other cyclists win with nutrition.

And finally, we are indebted to the many cycling organizations and individuals whose love of biking has inspired them to educate and advocate for safe, fun, and accessible riding.

WHEN MY FUTURE WIFE NANCY AND I BEGAN PREPARING FOR OUR FIRST LONG-distance bicycle tour in 1974, we knew as much about nutrition as we did about training for an epic tour. Which is to say, almost nothing.

We had begun planning our summer ride while still snow-bound at Grand Targhee Ski Resort in the Wyoming Tetons, where Nancy and I had serendipitously met after both landing jobs there for the winter. In truth, I probably should have known something about nutrition, because my job at the resort was that of head night cook for the restaurant. However, the only items on the menu that I had to prepare were grilled steaks, baked potatoes, deep-fried shrimp and chicken, and tossed salad. Prior to that, my culinary experience boiled down to having once baked a cherry cobbler in a Dutch oven for a Boy Scout merit badge.

Consequently, what ended up fueling us for the majority of the more than 2,000 miles we pedaled between Seattle and Rhinelander, Wisconsin, was peanut butter, bread, Coca Cola, and more peanut butter. When you're young and naturally energetic and don't know any better, you think you can get away with eating anything and do fine. I'm sure we would've done even better had we eaten properly, which we no doubt would have if a book like *The Cyclist's Food Guide* had been available to us at the time.

Whether training, racing, riding for fitness, or touring, every cyclist can benefit from a well-considered nutritional program. Keeping your fuel level up is important, but so too is the quality of the fuel you put in your tank. I've found in my experience as a road and mountain biker, 2:42 marathon runner, and Nordic skiing competitor (still going *somewhat* strong at age 53) that eating the right foods before, during, and after exercise improves performance and speeds up recovery. And you can't find any better advice on how to go about obtaining optimal nutrition than you'll glean by reading Nancy Clark and Jenny Hegmann's *The Cyclist's Food Guide*.

Nancy Clark is an internationally known sports nutritionist, a dedicated bike commuter, and a 1978 TransAmerica tour leader. Her popular column

"The Cyclists' Kitchen" is published in our association magazine, *Adventure Cyclist*, and she is also a regular contributor to *SHAPE* and *Runner's World* magazines. Nancy has counseled an array of athletes, ranging from first-time marathoners to members of the Boston Celtics basketball team. Jenny Hegmann, a registered dietitian specializing in sports nutrition, wellness, and weight management, is equally knowledgeable and passionate about providing nutritional advice for cyclists. Rarely a day goes by that Jenny is not on her bike—she commutes to work and has participated in randonnées, century rides, races, and weekend tours.

Nancy and Jenny insightfully impart their common-sense information on preventing fatigue during long rides, controlling winter weight gain, and ensuring proper protein intake on a vegetarian diet—and these are just a few tastes of what you'll find in *The Cyclist's Food Guide*. A cornucopia of information, the book brims with dietary details that are easy to understand and incorporate into your everyday life. You'll get more out of your cycling, be it fitness riding, racing, touring, even indoor spinning, by absorbing and adopting the sound basics contained within this book.

We are blessed at Adventure Cycling to have the opportunity to meet hundreds of fascinating bicyclists during their cross-country tours. They commonly talk about food, whether their journeys are powered primarily by gummy bears and potato chips or by more nutritious fare. Through stressing the hows and whys of eating right, The Cyclist's Food Guide contains the ingredients necessary to get these and all riders onto the road to high energy, good health, and smooth cycling.

—Michael McCoy

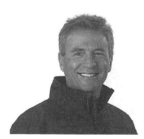

Michael McCoy has been involved with the Adventure Cycling Association (www.adventurecycling.org) since the organization began as Bikecentennial in the mid-1970s. Today he serves as field editor and staff writer, working from his home in Teton Valley, Idaho. His job is to help inspire people of all ages to travel by bicycle. Headquartered in Missoula, Montana, Adventure Cycling boasts over 41,000 members, and its National Bicycle Route Network encompasses more than 33,000 miles of roads perfectly suited for cycling.

JENNY AND I HAVE COVERED MANY MILES ON OUR BIKES OVER THE PAST 20 YEARS— commutes to work, century rides, transAmerica tours, randonnées, and races. As sports nutritionists, we have the advantage of knowing how to fuel our bodies for going and enjoying the distance.

Through our writing, counseling, and seminars, we have helped scores of active people achieve their goals with good nutrition. My best-selling *Nancy Clark's Sports Nutrition Guidebook*, now in its third edition, has been considered by many to be their sports nutrition bible. In *The Cyclist's Food Guide*, we combine our expertise in sports nutrition with our knowledge of cycling to deliver information that tells you how, what, and when to eat for optimal fueling and top performance.

Whether you are embarking on your first cycling adventure, your tenth tour, or your 100th race, we hope you will benefit from our practical, tried-and-true, and helpful advice. We provide ideas for easy meals, lists of foods, fluids, and nutrients, and tips from both coaches and experienced cyclists. Novice riders will find the words of wisdom they need to allay fears about running out of steam on the long rides and bonking on the hills. Seasoned riders, racers, and ultra-distance riders will find insight into sports supplements, timing of pre- and post-ride meals to enhance performance, and eating well despite long hours in the saddle.

When you put the information in *The Cyclist's Food Guide* into practice, you'll gain an edge over your peers who fuel their muscles poorly and fail to care for their health with premium nutrition.

We hope you make *The Cyclist's Food Guide* an integral part of your training program. It will answer your questions about nutrition for cycling, give you inspiration for the miles ahead, and help you fuel the distance strongly, whatever your cycling goals.

With best wishes for safe, smooth, and successful riding,

—*Nancy Clark, MS, RD and Jenny Hegmann, MS, RD*

The
CYCLIST'S
FOOD
GUIDE

FUELING FOR THE DISTANCE

CHAPTER 1

Your Daily Diet: What Shape Is It?

ARE YOU READY TO RIDE? YES, YOU'VE GOT YOUR HELMET AND BIKE... but is your body well—fueled with wholesome foods? Will your current diet support your biking goals? Are you nutritionally prepared? Due to the time constraints that riding imposes upon already busy schedules, many cyclists fail to plan for proper meals. They grab whatever is easy—this may be the same food day after day, month after month. Bagel for breakfast. Banana for snack. Pasta for dinner. Repetitive eating keeps life simple and minimizes decisions, but it can also take its toll: nutrient deficiencies, less-than-optimal athletic performance, and chronic fatigue.

This chapter reviews the basics of good nutrition for cyclists and will give you tips to make wise decisions about what you eat. Chapters 2 and 3 will give you ideas for quick and healthy breakfast, lunch, and dinner meals.

> **❝It's not just what I eat pre-ride and post-ride that impacts my riding and performance; It's my overall everyday diet. ❞**
>
> MaryAnn Martinez, Concord, MA

● **THE FOOD GUIDE PYRAMID**—If you eat a diet that lacks variety—for example, a steady diet of bagels, bananas, and pasta—you will chug along on a lackluster intake of vitamins, minerals, and other nutrients. It would be far better for you to reshape your flat diet into a well-rounded, nutritionally balanced diet, or better yet, a pyramid. The U.S. Department of Agriculture's model for healthy eating, the Food Guide Pyramid, reflects current knowledge on nutrition for good health. The three-dimensional pyramid suggests you should eat wholesome grain foods (preferably *whole*

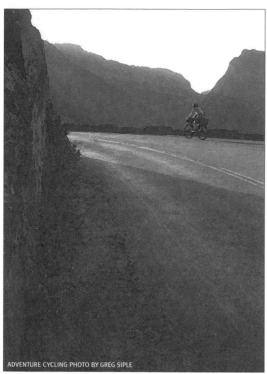

The food choices you make today will affect your performance, health, and ability to enjoy riding in the years to come, so choose wisely. Routinely eat healthful meals abundant with whole grains, fruits, and vegetables.

grains like brown rice, whole-wheat bread, oatmeal), fruits, and vegetables as the foundation of your diet. Lean animal proteins, plant proteins, and low-fat milk products should be included, but in lesser amounts. The tiny tip of the pyramid allows for fats, sweets, alcohol, and treats, if desired, but in moderation. Translated to meals, roughly three-quarters of your plate should be filled with whole grains, vegetables, and fruit and one-quarter of your plate with animal or vegetable protein and/or milk products. For a listing of a few of the most nutritious sports foods, refer to *Some Top Sports Foods* on page 3.

Not everyone understands the pyramid's messages of balance, variety, and moderation. Confusion abounds regarding the recommended number and sizes of food group servings, and how to fit them all into a day's menu:

Food group	*Number of recommended servings*
Grains	6-11
Fruits	2-4
Vegetables	3-5
Milk and milk foods	2-3
Protein-rich foods: meat, poultry, fish, legumes, eggs, and nuts	2-3
Total number of daily servings	= 15-26

Although 26 servings may sound like several five-course meals, the calories range from 1,600 to 2,800. This meets the needs of most people, including cyclists on short-ride or recovery days (see chapter 13: *Calculating Your Calorie Needs*). Recommended serving sizes are relatively small compared to today's super-size market and may be much smaller than what you are used to buying or being served in a restaurant.

Cyclists need not spend hours in the kitchen to have a healthful diet. The following foods offer top-quality nutrition and require little or no cooking.

Fruits

Citrus fruits are rich sources of vitamin C. Those with orange or yellow flesh are rich sources of beta-carotene, a precursor to vitamin A. Some top choices include:

- Oranges
- Grapefruit
- Tangerines
- Cantaloupe
- Strawberries
- Mango
- Kiwi
- Dried apricots

Vegetables

Vegetables need not be fresh to be nutritious; frozen or canned vegetables offer nutrition and convenience for the busy cyclist. For the most nutrients, choose dark green leafy vegetables and those that are orange, red, or bright yellow. Here are some good sources of beta-carotene and/or vitamin C:

- Broccoli
- Romaine and other dark green lettuces
- Spinach, collards, or kale
- Green, red, and yellow peppers
- Tomatoes
- Carrots
- Sweet potatoes
- Winter squash

Milk

Milk products offer a naturally good source of calcium:

- Low-fat or fat-free milk or flavored milk
- Low-fat or fat-free yogurt
- Reduced-fat cheese

Other sources of calcium include:

- Calcium-fortified orange juice, soymilk, and tofu

Meat and other proteins

Lean proteins that are quick and easy include:

- Deli roast beef, ham, and turkey
- Canned tuna and salmon
- Hummus
- Canned beans (such as refried beans or kidney beans)
- Nuts and nut butters: peanut, sunflower, almond
- Tofu
- Roasted soynuts
- Cottage cheese

Grains

Cook-free grains offer a convenient source of carbohydrates, B-vitamins, and fiber:

- High-fiber or whole-grain breakfast cereals (preferably iron-enriched)
- Low-fat granola or muesli
- Wholesome breads, rolls, and bagels
- Whole-wheat pita pockets, sandwich wraps, and tortillas
- Whole-grain crackers

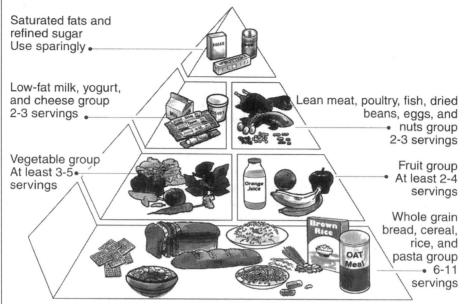

FOOD PYRAMID — A Guide to Daily Food Choices

Saturated fats and refined sugar
Use sparingly

Low-fat milk, yogurt, and cheese group
2-3 servings

Lean meat, poultry, fish, dried beans, eggs, and nuts group
2-3 servings

Vegetable group
At least 3-5 servings

Fruit group
At least 2-4 servings

Whole grain bread, cereal, rice, and pasta group
6-11 servings

Use the Food Guide Pyramid to help you eat a healthy sports diet every day. Choose plenty of whole-grain breads, cereals, rice, and pasta, and ample fruits and vegetables as the foundation of your daily diet. Enjoy two to three servings of low-fat or fat-free foods from the milk group and two to three servings of lean meat, poultry, fish, legumes, eggs, or nuts. Together, these food groups provide the nutrients you need. No single food group is more (or less) important than another—for good health, you need them all. Go easy on the fats, sweets, and alcohol in the small tip of the pyramid—these supply plenty of calories but little nutrition.

From N. Clark, Nancy Clark's Sports Nutrition Guidebook, 3rd ed, page 5. ©2003 by Nancy Clark. Reprinted with permission from Human Kinetics (Champaign, Il).

BALANCING YOUR DIET

The trick to getting the recommended servings of food groups each day is to balance them throughout your day. Plan to have at least three of the five food groups at each meal and one or two food groups at each snack. For example:

	Grain	Fruit	Vegetable	Milk	Meat/Protein
Breakfast:	cereal	banana	-----	milk	-----
Lunch:	bread	orange	vegetable soup	-----	peanut butter
Snack:	pretzels	-----	-----	yogurt	-----
Dinner:	spaghetti	-----	tomato sauce, broccoli	cheese	ground turkey
Snack:	popcorn	juice	-----	-----	-----

When selecting from the food groups, choose *wholesome* foods. Select minimally processed *whole grains*, which offer more nutrients and fiber and may have less added fat and sugar than their refined counterparts. For less saturated fat and cholesterol, have *low-fat* or *fat-free* milk, cheese, and yogurt; choose to eat more beans, nuts, fish, and lean poultry and less fatty meat. Opt for *colorful* fresh, frozen, or dried fruits and vegetables for the most nutrients.

● **CARBOHYDRATES FOR YOUR SPORTS DIET**—By eating fruits, vegetables, and grains as the foundation of each meal, you'll consume 55-65 percent of your calories from carbohydrates. This is exactly what you need for a high-energy sports diet. These are stored in muscles in the form of glycogen, the energy you need to train hard day after day, ride long distances, and compete well on race day.

Grain foods are a popular source of carbohydrates for active people. But even food-loving cyclists may balk at the recommendation to eat 6 to 11 servings of grains every day. To understand that this is a reasonable amount, you need to understand the definition of a "serving." A serving of grains is only 1 ounce (28 grams) dry weight or approximately ¹/₂ cup (120 milliliters) ready-to-eat and has about 75 calories. You should aim to have two to four servings (150 to 300 calories) of grains per meal, not much for hungry cyclists who require 600 to 900 calories at a meal. When possible, opt for whole grains rather than refined grains (shredded wheat instead of frosted flakes, whole-wheat bread instead of white) to give you more fiber and health-protective nutrients. Compare your serving sizes with those of the pyramid below:

Grains: Recommended Intake—6 to 11 Servings per Day			
Food	**Pyramid Serving Size**	**Cyclist's Usual Portion**	**# of Pyramid Servings**
Cold cereal	1 ounce	2–4 ounces (1 big bowl)	2–4
Hot oatmeal	½ cup cooked	1½ cups cooked	3
Bagel	½ small	1 large	3–4
Bread	1 slice	2 slices in sandwich	2
Pasta	½ cup cooked	2 cups cooked	4
Rice	½ cup cooked	1–2 cups cooked	2–4
1/2 cup = 120 milliliters; 1 ounce = 28 grams			

Fruits and vegetables are an excellent source of carbohydrates. They are like nature's vitamin pills, providing vitamin C, beta-carotene, fiber, and many other natural compounds that help maintain health and prevent disease. Research has repeatedly shown that diets rich in fruits and vegetables are protective against cancer, heart disease, and many other chronic health problems. But eating the recommended two to four servings of fruits and three to five servings of vegetables each day is another story. As one cyclist remarked, "I'm lucky if I eat that much in a week!" The trick is to eat large portions of them and to try to sneak them into your diet wherever possible—fruit in your morning cereal, dried fruit during a ride, or extra veggies in your lunchtime sandwich. For more ideas see *How to Eat More Vegetables*, on page 8.

● **PROTEIN FOR YOUR SPORTS DIET**—Like carbohydrates, protein-rich foods are an important part of your sports diet. If you follow the pyramid model, you will consume approximately 10-15 percent of your calories as protein, the recommended amount for a healthful sports diet. You should eat two to three servings each day from the protein group, bearing in mind that this group contains a variety of animal and non-animal foods (poultry, seafood, legumes, soymilk and tofu, nuts, and eggs).

Fruit: Recommended Intake—2 to 4 Servings per Day (2 cups or more)			
Food	**Pyramid Serving Size**	**Cyclist's Usual Portion**	**# of Pyramid Servings**
Orange juice	6 ounces	12 ounces	2
Apple, orange peach, or pear	1 medium	1 large	2
Banana	1 small	1 large	2
Fruit Salad	½ cup	1 cup	2

Vegetables: Recommended Intake—3 to 5 Servings per Day (2.5 cups or more)			
Food	**Pyramid Serving Size**	**Cyclist's Usual Portion**	**# of Pyramid Servings**
Broccoli	1 small stalk	2 large stalks	3–4
Carrots, peas	½ cup, cooked	1 cup	2
Salad greens	1 cup	1 large bowl	3–4
Spaghetti sauce	½ cup	1 cup	2

1 cup = 240 millititers; 6 ounces = 180 millititers

Cyclists tend to either over- or underconsume protein. Some fill up on animal proteins like big burgers, slabs of steaks, eggs (or egg whites), and chicken, and get more than enough protein (and often, way too much saturated fat). Others bypass these foods in their efforts to eat a low-fat, meat-free, or vegetarian diet, but neglect to eat adequate non-animal sources of protein, such as beans and tofu, resulting in a protein-deficient diet. For additional information and more specific guidelines on protein see chapter 5. Compare your protein intake to the recommended intake:

Proteins: Recommended Intake—2 to 3 Servings per Day			
Food	Pyramid Serving Size	Cyclist's Usual Portion	# of Pyramid Servings
Tuna, canned	⅓ of a 6-ounce can	1 whole can	3
Chicken	1 leg	1 breast	3
Peanut butter	2 tablespoons	2 – 4 tablespoons	1–2
Lentil or bean soup	1 cup	1 bowl	2
Kidney beans	½ cup	1 cup	2
1 cup = 240 milliliters; 1 tablespoon = 15 milliliters; 1 ounce = 28 grams			

To fully meet your protein and nutrition needs you should also consume 2 to 3 servings of calcium-rich milk products, such as low-fat milk, yogurt, and cheese (or other calcium-rich foods, such as calcium-fortified soymilk). Getting enough calcium is necessary to maximize bone health and bone density, a particular concern for growing teens and women. Research shows that consuming calcium-rich foods may also play a role in facilitating weight loss and protecting against high blood pressure. For only 300 to 400 calories, you can meet 100 percent of your daily calcium requirement by eating:
- 8 ounces (240 milliliters) of low-fat milk or fortified soymilk on breakfast cereal plus
- 8 ounces (240 milliliters) of low-fat milk or fortified soymilk with lunch plus
- 8 ounces (240 milliliters) of low-fat yogurt or 1¹/₂ ounces (42 grams) or reduced-fat cheese for a snack.

Note that fat-free and low-fat products are preferable for heart health and calorie control, but you need not suffer with

Cyclists who live alone, work long hours, don't cook or cook very little, and/or eat primarily fast foods commonly have vegetable-poor diets. Most of them know that they should eat more vegetables, but they have a difficult time fitting them into their diets. Even if they make the time to shop and stock their fridge with vegetables, they may not be home often enough to cook and eat them before they go bad. If getting your three to five servings of vegetables a day is a constant struggle, the following tips may help you to enhance your nutritional status.

- *Eat more of the best, less of the rest.* In general, dark green, deep yellow, orange, and red vegetables have far more nutrients than those that are pale. Hence, if you dislike pale zucchini, celery, and green beans, don't work hard to acquire a taste for them. Instead, put your efforts into having more colorful choices: broccoli, spinach, romaine lettuce, winter squash, tomatoes, and carrots.
- *Eat colorful salads.* Salad bars at supermarkets and restaurants are easy ways to get your quota of vegetables, but choose carefully. Fill your bowl with tomatoes, red and green peppers, carrots, and dark lettuces and use low-fat or fat-free dressing. Avoid pale salads with white lettuce, cucumbers, mushrooms, celery, and other lack-luster veggies that offer little more than crunch, and oily dressings, which simply coat the crunch with grease, a far cry from good nutrition. You'd be better off choosing tomato juice, vegetable soups (even canned soups are better than nothing), or a handful of raw baby carrots for a pre-dinner appetizer.
- *Fortify spaghetti sauce and soups with extra vegetables.* Simply add a box of frozen chopped broccoli or spinach or a handful of frozen mixed vegetables to your favorite pasta sauce or canned soup and heat as usual. If using fresh vegetables, simply cook them separately—in a steamer over the pasta water, in a covered saucepan with one-half inch of water, or in a covered dish in the microwave—until tender, then add to the sauce or soup.

fat-free milk if you really don't like it. You can always cut back on fat in other foods in your diet. For example, have fat-free salad dressing or skip the butter on your dinner potato. For more information on dietary fat, see chapter 6.

Those who prefer a dairy-free diet or are lactose intolerant should take special care to eat adequate amounts of lactose-free or nondairy calcium sources. See *Calcium Equivalents* on page 10 for suggestions.

● **THE TIP OF THE PYRAMID: FATS, OILS, AND SWEETS**—Despite recommendations to eat a healthful diet based on grains, fruits,

- *Choose fast foods with the most veggies:*
  - Pizza with peppers, mushrooms, and extra tomato sauce
  - Chinese or Asian entrées stir-fried with vegetables
  - Lunchtime V-8 juice instead of diet soda
  - Subs, sandwiches, or roll-ups with less meat and extra lettuce and tomato
  - Salad entrée or side salad with reduced-fat dressing with your sandwich
- *Even over-cooked vegetables are better than no vegetables.* If your only option is over-cooked veggies from the cafeteria, eat them. Cooking destroys some nutrients but not all of them. Any vegetable is better than no vegetable!
- *Keep frozen vegetables stocked in your freezer.* Then you'll always have vegetables on hand, ready to go. They are quick and easy to prepare (they are pre-washed and pre-cut), stay fresh for weeks, and have far more nutrients than "fresh" vegetables that have been in the store and your refrigerator for several days.
- *Maximize your nutrient intake by cooking vegetables properly.* Cooking reduces a vegetable's nutritional content, so:
  - Quickly steam vegetables only until tender crisp, using very little water, and use the cooking water as a broth.
  - Microwave vegetables in a covered dish with little or no water.
  - Stir-fry vegetables with very little oil.
- *When all else fails, eat fruit to help compensate for a lack of vegetables.* The best alternatives include bananas, oranges, grapefruit, cantaloupe, strawberries, mango, and kiwi. These choices are rich in many of the same nutrients found in vegetables.

and vegetables, some cyclists eat too many calories from fats, oils, and sweets. If you have a junk-food diet that topples your pyramid, you can correct this imbalance by eating larger breakfasts and lunches with wholesome foods from the base and body of the pyramid before you get too hungry. Cyclists who get too hungry crave and tend to choose foods high in fats and refined sugar (e.g. candy, cookies, chips) from the tip of the pyramid. The simple solution to the junk-food diet is to prevent hunger and sweet cravings by eating satisfying, nourishing meals regularly throughout the day and by appropriately fueling before, during, and after rides (see chapters 8, 9, and 10).

The recommended daily calcium intake is:

Age Group	Calcium (milligrams)
Teens, 9–18 years	1,300
Adults, 19–50 years	1,000
Adults, 51+ years	1,200

Source: Dietary Reference Intakes, National Academy of Science

The following foods all provide about 300 milligrams of calcium. Two to three choices per day, or one at each meal, will contribute to meeting your calcium needs.

Calcium-rich Food	Amount
Milk	
Milk	1 cup
Yogurt	1 cup
Cheese	1½ ounces
Cottage cheese	2 cups
Frozen yogurt	1½ cups

Calcium-rich Food	Amount
Vegetable	
Broccoli, cooked	3 cups
Collard or turnip greens, cooked	1 cup
Kale or mustard greens, cooked	1½ cups
Protein	
Soymilk	1 cup
Tofu (½ cake)	5 ounces
Salmon, canned with bones	4 ounces
Sardines, canned with bones	2½ ounces
Almonds	¾ cup

1 cup = 240 millititers
1 ounce = 28 grams

> **One of my favorite recovery foods is a baked sweet potato topped with a few raisins and a little brown sugar. I pre-bake them and keep a stash in the refrigerator so I can simply reheat and eat.**
>
> Louise Wilcox, Reading, MA

The inclusion of fats and sweets in the tip of the pyramid suggests that you do not need to eat a perfect diet (i.e. no fat, no sugar, no fun!) to have a good diet. Yes, you can enjoy a cookie for dessert after having eaten a sandwich, milk, and fruit for lunch. But don't eat cookies for lunch and skip the sandwich. That's when nutrition and performance problems arise. To key to balancing fats and sugars appropriately in your diet is to abide by these guidelines:

- 10 percent of your calories can appropriately come from refined sugar (200–300 calories or 50-75 grams of refined sugar per day for most cyclists)
- 25 percent of your calories can appropriately come from fat (500–750 calories or 55–85 grams of fat per day for most cyclists)

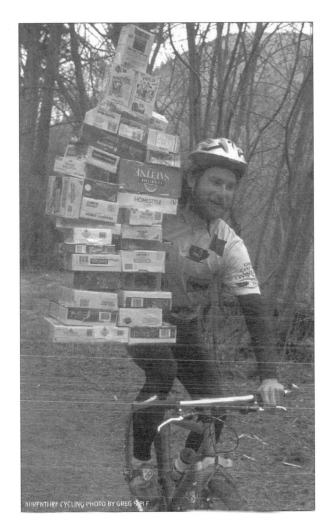

ADVENTURE CYCLING PHOTO BY GREG SIPLE

> **❝I try to live by the 80/20 rule: 80 percent of the time I eat nutritious food; 20 percent of the time I have fun foods as a reward for my hard training. The 20 percent includes chocolate, beer, onion rings, blue cheese, doughnuts, and ice cream. ❞**
>
> Earl Fenstermacher, Seattle, WA

Hence, moderate amounts of chips, salad dressing, jam, and cookies can nourish you with a livable and tasty food plan.

● WANT SOME HELP SHAPING UP YOUR DIET?—

If you want personalized dietary advice, we recommend that you have a nutrition checkup with a registered dietitian who specializes in sports nutrition. To find one in your area, call at (800) 366-1655 or visit the American Dietetic Association's referral network on their website at www.eatright.org. You'll be glad you did!

> **❝My favorite breakfast is hot oatmeal with a spoonful of canned pumpkin or frozen berries, and a dash of cinnamon and brown sugar. It tastes great and I get a jump on my fruit and vegetable intake before 8 a.m. ❞**
>
> Paul Humphries, Reading, MA

- **SUMMARY**—As a cyclist, your nutritional fitness is as important as your physical fitness.
- The food pyramid suggests you should eat wholesome grain foods, fruits, and vegetables as the foundation of your diet with lesser amounts of milk and protein foods and just a sprinkling of fats, oils, and sweets.
- By eating according to the pyramid, you'll consume 55-65 percent of your calories from carbohydrates and 10-15 percent of your calories from protein, the ideal sports diet for an active cyclist.
- Make wise choices on a daily basis by choosing minimally processed whole grains, colorful fruits and vegetables, low-fat or fat-free milk products, and more beans, fish, and lean poultry and less fatty meat.
- Improve a vegetable-poor diet by choosing the most nutritious vegetables, eating larger portions of them, and incorporating them into sandwiches, soups, and pasta.

CHAPTER 2

Breakfast: The Meal of Champions

GOOD NUTRITION FOR CYCLISTS STARTS AT BREAKFAST. THIS IS THE most important meal of the day because it fuels your body and mind for a day of high energy and healthful eating. Yet many cyclists skip breakfast. They push themselves through their busy schedules and struggle with low energy, less-than-stellar riding, cravings for fatty sweets, hunger, and often unwanted weight gain. If you are a breakfast skipper, consider the following:

- Breakfast eaters consume a more healthful diet that has more fiber, calcium, iron, and whole grains and less dietary fat than do breakfast skippers. As a result, they have a reduced risk of osteoporosis, heart disease, and anemia.
- Eating breakfast raises morning-low blood sugar levels and improves wakefulness, mood, concentration, and productivity.
- Breakfast gives you a leg-up on calories for your active day, tops off depleted glycogen stores, and gives you the energy and power to ride and work hard.
- Breakfast eaters are more successful with weight control.

- **EXCUSES, EXCUSES**—If breakfast is so good for us, then why do so many people skip it? There are plenty of excuses: no time, too busy, not hungry,

> **" Breakfast is not my favorite meal of the day, but I soon learned it was essential to my overall endurance. My training sessions and times were markedly worse when I skipped breakfast. A bagel or cereal in the morning works wonders for me! "**
>
> Shelley Smith,
> Highlands Ranch, CO

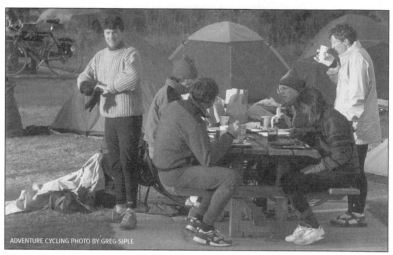

Enjoying a wholesome breakfast with friends is one of the pleasures of bike touring. For all cyclists, breakfast provides fuel for more energy and stronger riding.

> **❝When my legs feel like mud, I know I didn't eat enough breakfast.❞**
>
> **Rich Lesnik, San Francisco, CA**

you name it. But for every excuse to skip breakfast there is an even better reason not to.

Excuse: "I don't have time." If you have no time for breakfast, keep in mind that you can always make time to do what you *want* to do. A lack of priority may be the real problem, not a lack of time. Breakfast need not be elaborate. You can prepare and eat breakfast in mere minutes whether at home, at a campsite, or on the run:

- Get up ten minutes earlier to eat a bowl of cereal.
- Munch on a bagel and juice as you break camp.
- Enjoy leftover pizza as you get dressed.
- Sip on milk and juice or a smoothie as you drive to work.

Here are a few quick, grab-and-go items for a healthy breakfast:

- Raisins or dried apricots and dry cereal tossed into a plastic bag
- Pita pocket with two slices of reduced-fat cheese
- A carton of fruit-flavored cottage cheese or yogurt
- Apple, orange, or banana plus a handful of crackers, nuts, or dry cereal
- Packets of instant oatmeal with an individual box of raisins
- Individual cartons of juice and milk or soymilk
- Toasted mini waffles, sandwiched with peanut butter

The key to breakfast during the morning rush is to plan

Not everyone likes cereal, pancakes, or bagels, but don't let that be a reason to skip breakfast. Choose foods you enjoy, even if it's last night's leftovers. After all, you are more likely to eat breakfast if it tastes good. Remember, eating any food in the morning is better than eating nothing!

Some suggestions:

- Peanut butter and banana on graham crackers
- Tomato, vegetable, or split pea soup
- Microwaved "baked" potato topped with cheese
- Tuna, turkey, or peanut butter sandwich
- Cheese (reduced-fat) and crackers
- Veggie burger on a bun
- Macaroni and cheese
- Leftover spaghetti, tuna-noodle casserole, or lasagna
- Cold pizza or leftover Chinese food

ahead. When touring, go food shopping the prior evening and stock up on breakfast staples. At home, prepare your breakfast the night before so you have it in a hurry: pour a bowl of cereal so all you have to do is add milk; set out the peanut butter jar and a sliced bagel; or pack a brown bag with yogurt and fruit and keep it in the refrigerator. It can be helpful to slice bagels, muffins, and rolls and store the slices in individual bags in the freezer; simply take one or two out of the freezer at night so breakfast is ready and waiting in the morning.

Excuse: "Breakfast interferes with my training schedule." If you are an early morning rider, you will perform better and avoid an energy crash if you eat something beforehand. Coffee with extra milk, a swig of juice, and a bagel or toast contributes to greater stamina and helps you feel more awake. If you have trouble tolerating early-morning, pre-ride food, try consuming just a simple snack of easy-to-digest foods, such as a half-slice of toast with jelly and a small glass of juice, or a handful of cereal with fat-free milk. If you can tolerate no food, eat a hefty snack the night before, such as a sandwich, bagel, or a large bowl of cereal.

Breakfast is equally important if you ride mid-day or in the afternoon. Eating breakfast tops off depleted glycogen stores and increases energy reserves to fuel mind and body during exercise.

If you train both in the morning and in the afternoon, eat breakfast before and after your morning workout (that is, two breakfasts). Because your muscles absorb the most carbohydrate within the first two hours after hard exercise, a quick and easy recovery breakfast is essential for a strong second workout.

Excuse: "I'm not hungry in the morning." If you have no morning appetite, the chances are you ate your breakfast calories the night before. Did you eat a huge dinner, lots of ice cream, or a big snack before bedtime? The solution to having no morning appetite is to eat less at night so you can start the day off hungry.

Some people find that training hard first thing in the morning kills their appetite. This lack of hunger is due to the rise in body temperature. Appetite should return within an hour or healthful choices. Sugar grams on current nutrition labels do not differentiate sugars that are added to make a food sweet—refined sugars, such as granulated sugar and corn syrup—from those that occur naturally, such as lactose in milk and fructose in raisins. Check the *ingredient* list to determine if a cereal has added sugars or not. Ingredients are listed in order by weight from most to least. Sugar, corn syrup, honey, sucrose, fructose, and other added sweeteners should not be among the first few ingredients. Choose those with whole wheat, brown rice, corn, or oats as the top ingredients.

Sugar is a carbohydrate that fuels muscles, but it lacks nutrients for good health. Ten percent of daily calories can appropriately come from added sugar; each gram of sugar provides four calories. Someone who eats 2,400 calories a day can have 240 calories, or 60 grams, of added sugar a day. To put this in perspective, the amount of sugar in Honey-Nut Cheerios (10 grams of sugar per one-cup serving) is relatively small compared to amount of sugar in other sweet foods, such as cola (40 grams of sugar per 12-ounce can) or M&Ms (30 grams of sugar per 1.6-ounce package). Obviously, the Cheerios, though sweetened with some added sugar, offers far more protein, fiber, and other nutrients than the cola or chocolate.

4. *Choose low-fat cereals with two grams of fat or less per serving.*

Eating a high-fat diet can contribute excess calories that lead to weight gain. Diets rich in saturated and trans fat are associated with cardiovascular disease. Some brands of cereals, particularly granola, can add unexpected fat and calories to your sports diet. Select low-fat brands for the foundation of your breakfast, and then use only a sprinkling of the higher-fat cereals, if desired, for a topping. See chapter 6 for more information about fat.

two after the body cools down. Plan ahead, so that when hunger hits there are healthful foods ready and waiting. Otherwise, you are likely to grab whatever is easy, which may include doughnuts, pastries, cookies, and other high-fat foods with little nutritional value.

Excuse: "I'm on a diet." Too many weight-conscious cyclists start their diet at breakfast. Bad idea. People who skip breakfast tend to gain weight and be heavier than people who eat breakfast. Eating a satisfying breakfast prevents you from becoming overly hungry and overeating. Breakfast gives you the energy to ride harder and longer so you burn more calories and improve your physical condition.

Many breakfast skippers believe they will eat more calories

and gain weight if they eat breakfast. Consider this: People who skip breakfast eat the majority of their day's calories at dinner and before bedtime. They eat dinner yet complain of having the "munchies" all evening; they end up snacking, often on large amounts of sweets, ice cream, or chips until bedtime. A hungry cyclist can easily consume over half a day's worth of calories this way. If this sounds familiar, you would be better off shifting some of those evening calories to a bigger breakfast and lunch. You'll have more energy when you need it most, during the day and during your ride. You'll be less hungry in the evening so you can eat a sensible dinner and avoid the post-dinner munchies that can ruin a sports diet. Chapter 14 has more details about how to lose weight and have energy to train.

Excuse: *"Breakfast makes me hungrier."* Some cyclists complain that if they eat breakfast, they are more hungry and eat more all day. This may result from thinking they have already "blown" their diets by eating breakfast, so they might as well keep overeating and then start dieting again the next day. Wrong. If you feel hungry after breakfast, you probably ate too little. One hundred calories of toast with jam merely whets your appetite and does not satisfy your calorie needs. You should budget one-third of your daily calories for your morning meal(s). A 150-pound (70-kilogram) cyclist who rides an hour a day may need 800 to 900 calories in the morning, the equivalent of three slices of toast with jam, a large glass of juice, eight ounces (240 milliliters) of low-fat yogurt, and a banana. If that is too much food for you to eat in one sitting, split it in half and enjoy two smaller breakfasts—eat a first breakfast a 7 a.m. and a second breakfast at 9:30 a.m. It is far better to consume your calories during the day when your body needs them than to wait until evening when you are winding down for the night. If you eat enough at breakfast you will not be as hungry for lunch and dinner and will be able to eat smaller portions. See chapter 13 for more information on how to calculate your calorie needs.

● **THE BREAKFAST OF CHAMPIONS**—By now we hope we have convinced you that breakfast is indeed the most important meal of the day. What is best to eat, you wonder? As a general rule, you should choose foods from at least three of the five food groups (such as grain + milk + fruit). We highly recommend a whole-some cereal as the breakfast of champions for several reasons. Cereal is:

- *Nutritious.* A bowl of cereal with fruit and milk supplies three of the five food groups and supplies calcium, fiber, and other nutrients active people need. Iron-fortified cereals provide a source of iron to help reduce your risk of becoming anemic.
- *Carbohydrate-rich.* Your brain and muscles need carbohydrates to work well. A bowl of cereal with milk and banana supplies you with three good sources of carbohydrates.
- *Quick, easy, and portable.* With cereal in your kitchen cupboard, desk drawer, pannier, or travel bag, you will always have a no-mess, no-cook, high-carbohydrate meal or snack to eat.
- *Versatile.* You can eat it dry if you're on the run or preferably, with low-fat milk or yogurt for a protein and calcium booster. You can have it not only for breakfast but also for a snack. You can mix brands and vary the flavor with different toppings:
  - Yogurt or soymilk instead of milk
  - Chopped dates or dried apricots
  - Dried cranberries and sunflower seeds
  - Brown sugar or maple syrup
  - Sliced fresh apple or peach
  - Walnuts, cinnamon, and sliced banana
  - Peanut or almond butter and cinnamon (for hot cereal)
  - Applesauce and brown sugar (for hot cereal)
  - Pumpkin (canned), cinnamon, and brown sugar (for hot cereal)
  - Frozen berries: Nancy's favorite is to put a mix of cereals in a bowl, top it with frozen blueberries, heat it in the microwave oven for 30 to 60 seconds, and then add cold milk. It is like eating fruit cobbler!

> **"My pre-ride/race breakfast food is the same 99 percent of the time: a bowl of homemade Irish oatmeal with maple syrup, cinnamon, and soymilk. I eat a substantial second breakfast right after my workout, usually a banana, a bagel with peanut butter, and a coffee with soymilk. "**
>
> MaryAnn Martinez, Concord, MA

Note that you should choose your cereals carefully. Some varieties are largely refined flour with lots of extra sugar and fat. To help you choose the best breakfast cereals, see page 16. Other good choices include wholesome carbohydrate-rich foods, such as whole-grain bagels, hot or cold cereals, pancakes, whole-wheat toast, fresh fruit, low-fat yogurt and milk, and low-fat bran muffins. Greasy bacon-and-egg meals or low-carb, egg white-and-veggie omelets lack the carbohydrates you need to optimally fuel your muscles with glycogen. Of course, eating *anything*, even a bowl of frozen yogurt or a couple of cookies, is better than eating nothing.

● **SUMMARY**—Simply put, eat breakfast. The best choices for breakfast include wholesome carbohydrate-based foods such as cereal with milk, fruit, and bagels. But remember, eating or drinking anything is better than nothing.
- Food in the morning provides fuel for more energy and stronger workouts, essential for improving your fitness level and cycling performance.
- Dieters can enjoy breakfast without the fear of sabotaging their diets. Breakfast curbs evening appetite so dieters can eat lighter at night.
- If you generally skip breakfast, at least give breakfast a try on the days you ride. You'll soon learn why breakfast is the meal of champions! See chapter 8 for more on the importance of pre-ride food.

CHAPTER 3

Lunch, Snacks, and Dinner

CYCLISTS SHOULD BE IN THE CONTINUOUS CYCLE OF FUELING AND refueling so that they have the energy to perform their best at work and at play. Starting the day with a substantial breakfast and following up with snacks, lunch, and dinner is essential.

Rule of Thumb for Healthful Meals—Given that lunch, snacks, and dinner supply the majority of your day's calories, you should wisely choose these foods to assure you are getting the optimal sports diet. A good rule of thumb for meals is to choose foods from at least three of the five food groups; for snacks, choose from two food groups. For example:

- *Lunch:* turkey sandwich and an apple
  (protein + grain + fruit)
- *Snack:* graham crackers with peanut butter
  (grain + protein)
- *Dinner:* spaghetti with tomato sauce, meatballs, and a glass of milk
  (grain + vegetable + protein + milk)

Because good nutrition starts in the supermarket, you have a far better chance of achieving a super sports diet when your kitchen is well-stocked with appropriate foods. You might want to make a copy of the *Cyclist's Basic Shopping List* (page 22) and post it on your refrigerator.

> **❝I usually spend one day a week shopping and preparing a lot of food. I cut up and wash all the fruits and vegetables, cook some chicken, and even boil and prepare pasta for the week. It saves so much time. ❞**
> Kate Riedell, Fairfield, CT

Cupboard:
- hot and cold cereal
- spaghetti (whole-wheat or regular)
- egg noodles
- spaghetti sauce
- brown rice
- crackers
- kidney beans
- baked beans
- refried beans
- peanut butter
- soups (mushroom for making casseroles, lentil, minestrone, hearty bean)
- V-8 or other 100% vegetable juices
- raisins
- dried apricots or apples, nonperishable snack foods (see page 29 *Some Super Sport Snacks*)
- canned salmon
- sardines
- tuna
- olive oil and canola oil
- your favorite seasonings (garlic, cinnamon, soy sauce, etc.)
- nuts

Countertop:
- bananas
- tomatoes
- oranges
- russet and sweet potatoes (for baking)
- onions

Refrigerator:
- reduced-fat cheese
- low-fat cottage cheese
- low-fat milk
- soymilk
- low-fat yogurt
- parmesan cheese
- eggs
- tofu
- tempeh
- flour and corn tortillas
- salad fixings
- carrots
- Romaine lettuce
- apples
- grapes
- hummus
- salsa
- 100% fruit juices
- sliced deli turkey and lean roast beef
- salsa
- reduced-fat salad dressing
- reduced-fat mayonnaise
- your favorite condiments (mustard, jellies, ketchup, etc.)

Freezer:
- whole-grain bagels
- whole-wheat pita
- English muffins
- multigrain bread and hamburger buns
- low-fat bran muffins
- orange juice concentrate
- broccoli
- spinach
- winter squash

- peas
- corn
- blueberries or other fruit
- ground turkey
- extra-lean hamburger
- chicken (pieces frozen individually)
- seafood
- veggie or soy burgers

Menu Ideas:
If you keep these food stocked in your kitchen, you will have the makings for at least a week of simple, carbohydrate-based meals:
- Pasta with tomato and meat, seafood, or beans
- Quick stirfry
- Easy casseroles like tuna or chicken noodle
- Homemade pizzas
- A variety of soups and hot or cold sandwiches
- Meat or vegetarian burritos or tacos
- Baked potatoes with your choice of hearty toppings
- Meal-sized salads with veggies, pasta, and protein
- Hearty hot or cold sandwiches

● **KNOWING WHEN TO EAT**—You should plan to eat at least every four hours throughout the day based on your hunger and physical desire to eat. While touring, you'll want to eat at least every two hours. Many cyclists go too long between meals; they routinely ignore hunger and put off eating for hours because it is not the standard time to eat. They may be hungry by 10 a.m. yet they wait to eat until "lunchtime" at noon. Sound familiar? If you are hungry, you shouldn't wait to eat. After all, hunger is simply your body's request for more fuel. Denying your hunger can lead to extreme hunger and then overeating, sweet cravings, and lags in energy. As an active cyclist, you can expect to get hungry every two to four hours, and you should plan your meals accordingly. If you eat breakfast at 7 a.m., you can appropriately be hungry for a first lunch at 10 a.m. and then a second lunch at 2 p.m.—with a few snacks in between, if you are on the road.

You also should take care to distribute your day's calories evenly among your meals. Each meal or section of the day—morning, noon, and evening—should provide you with approximately the same number of calories. Lots of cyclists and other active people eat too little at their daytime meals, only to consume most of their day's calorie budget after 5 p.m. But why wait until evening to eat when those calories could be used to energize your day and your workout? If you generally wait until the end of your day to enjoy the majority of your day's calories, you may want to rethink your eating plan. Here are two examples for someone who needs 2,400 calories a day:

> **For our honeymoon, we biked from Holland to Greece. We enjoyed eating much of our food from local markets and eateries along the route—plenty of delicious fresh bread, pasta, meats, and fruit. In Europe, places typically are closed from noon to 2 p.m., so we quickly learned to plan our meals around that!**
>
> Skip and Danielle Komisar, Cheshire, CT

Four Meals a Day

Meal	Time	Calories
Breakfast	7 a.m.	600
First lunch	10 a.m.	600
Second lunch	2 p.m.	600
Dinner	6 p.m.	600

Five Meals a Day

Meal	Time	Calories
Breakfast	7 a.m.	600
Snack	10 a.m.	300
Lunch	1 p.m.	600
Snack	4 p.m.	300
Dinner	7 p.m.	600

● **LUNCH**—Whereas breakfast is the most important meal of the day, lunch is the second most important. Breakfast fills your tank with fuel; lunch replenishes it. Lunch renews glycogen stores drained by morning activities and provides fuel for the afternoon. Cyclists who skip or skimp on lunch compromise their training, and their enjoyment of training, by:

• not being properly fueled for the afternoon or evening workout,

• getting overly hungry and gorging on goodies all evening, and

• missing out on the nutrients muscles need to recover from the morning workout.

Brown Bagging It—If you are organized enough to do it, making your own lunch and bringing it with you is the best option for many reasons. It saves money (you don't have to order out), saves time (you don't have to head to the cafeteria), and can be more nutritious compared to high-fat restaurant food. The key is to make lunch preparation fast and simple. See Brown-Bag Lunches, on page 25 for helpful tips.

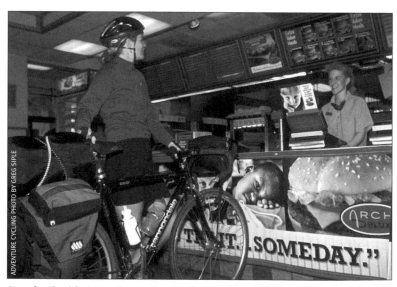

Does fast food fuel your day, or does it ruin your sports diet? When you are on the road or can't pack your own wholesome lunch, quick-service restaurants and convenience stores can provide a healthful meal, if you choose wisely.

● BROWN-BAG LUNCHES

The following suggestions may help you pack a super sports lunch.

- Make lunch the night before to reduce chaos in your morning rush hour.

- To keep sandwich bread fresh, store it in the freezer and take out the slices as needed. Bread thaws in minutes at room temperature or in seconds in the microwave oven.

- Make several sandwiches at once and store them in the freezer. Grab one on your way out the door. The frozen sandwich will be thawed and fresh by lunchtime. Sliced meats and peanut butter freeze nicely. Don't freeze eggs, mayonnaise, or raw vegetables.

- Try different low-fat sandwich spreads: low-fat or fat-free mayonnaise, plain yogurt or yogurt/mayonnaise mixtures, low-fat or fat-free salad dressings, honey-mustard, salsa, or hummus.

- Add a good helping of lettuce and tomato to a sandwich for a full serving of vegetables.

- Buy pre-washed fresh vegetables, such as peeled baby carrots, salad, broccoli florets, shredded cabbage, coleslaw mix, and carrots to save time and hassle. Toss a variety together for a quick salad or add them to sandwiches, roll-ups, or pita pockets.

- Liven up an old fashioned peanut butter sandwich by adding sliced banana or apple, raisins, or dates.

- Slice low-fat cheese, store it in a sealed container or plastic bag, and keep it in the refrigerator. Make a meat-free sandwich with cheese, peppers, avocado, and sprouts.

- Keep a tub of hummus in the refrigerator and a package of lavash, pita bread, or flour tortillas in the freezer. Thaw the bread or tortilla in the microwave, add hummus and a combination of pre-washed raw vegetables, and roll it up for a tasty vegetarian wrap.

- Keep a bowl of fresh fruit, like bananas, oranges, and washed apples, pears, and plums, on the kitchen counter or in your desk at work for easy access.

- Stock up on individual containers of yogurt, cottage cheese, canned fruit, pudding, 100% fruit and vegetable juices, and string cheese to toss in your lunch bag.

- At dinner, always cook extra so you have leftovers for tomorrow's lunch. Distribute the food among a few small microwaveable containers, making several complete meals, and store them in the refrigerator or freezer. This way, a balanced meal of soup, chili, pasta, or meat and potatoes is on hand for you to grab and go.

Fast-Food Meals—Unfortunately, few cyclists make the effort to organize their lunch plans in advance of noontime. If that describes you, fast food can save the day, or it can spoil your sports diet. The traditional fast-food meal is loaded with fat, sodium, and cholesterol and is low in fiber. The good news is that most quick-service restaurants now offer healthful options: low-fat chicken sandwiches, hearty soups, salads, and even vegetarian burgers. Though you may be tempted to order a deluxe burger and fries, remind yourself that you will be healthier, feel better, and feel better about yourself if you forgo the grease and order the healthful option. Below are suggestions for lower-fat meals found at popular quick-service restaurants.

Dunkin' Donuts:	Reduced-fat or fat-free muffin or bagel, and a cup of bean or broth-based soup; egg on a bagel or English muffin
McDonald's:	Chicken McGrill or hamburger, side salad, and vanilla reduced-fat ice cream cone or Fruit'n Yogurt Parfait
Burger King:	Grilled Chicken Baguette, BK Veggie Burger, hamburger, or chili, plus a side salad
Wendy's:	Chili without cheese and a baked potato; hamburger or grilled chicken sandwich and a side salad; Mandarin Chicken Salad and a baked potato; a Jr. Frosty for dessert
Taco Bell:	Plain bean burrito or soft chicken taco with extra lettuce and tomato. Limit cheese and sour cream.
Pizza:	Cheese slice with extra veggies rather than extra cheese, pepperoni, or 'stuffed' varieties
Subway:	Turkey, ham, or roast beef sub on a whole-grain roll and loaded with fresh vegetables; broth-based soup plus a whole grain roll
Pasta:	Spaghetti with tomato sauce, plain or with grilled chicken or meatballs
Asian:	Hot and sour, wonton, or noodle soups; steamed rice with stir-fried entrée such as beef and broccoli or chicken with vegetable (request the food be cooked with minimal oil); sushi; fresh spring rolls (not fried)

Sandwich, bagel, *or sub shop*	Turkey, ham, roast beef, or grilled chicken on whole-wheat roll, bagel, or bread plus extra lettuce and tomato; vegetable, bean, or broth-based soup, side salad, and sub roll.
Beverages *and condiments*	Most quick-service restaurants carry low-fat milk, fruit juice, tomato juice, and hot chocolate. These are far more nutritious than soda pop, lemonade, iced tea, or sugary coffee drinks. At restaurants that serve salads, choose low-fat or reduced-fat dressings.

• **SNACKS**—In many countries such as England or Germany, it is traditional to enjoy an afternoon cup of coffee or tea along with a sweet. This scheduled snack provides a pleasant break as well as an energy booster. In comparison, many Americans believe eating between meals is sinful. If they succumb, they feel guilty.

One reason why people think snacking is bad is because they snack on candy, cookies, doughnuts, or chips. These foods provide few nutrients needed for optimal cycling performance. A better choice is to trade 250 calories of candy bar for 250 calories of nuts and raisins. Appropriate snacking refuels you, gives you necessary nutrients, and gives you extra energy to perform your best on the bike. It can be good for you and should be a part of your training and touring diet.

The Four O'clock Munchies—As we have said, hunger is not bad or wrong and is merely your body's request for fuel. It is a normal physiological request that comes every three to four hours. So even if you eat breakfast at 8 a.m. and lunch at noon, you are likely to feel hungry, or have the munchies, in the afternoon. If you fight your afternoon hunger and forgo this important snack, you may find that you suffer from:

• *Uncontrollable sweet cravings*—If you crave and nibble on sweets constantly you may

> **Recently, I went on a group ride that started at noon so I chose not to eat lunch, fearing I wouldn't feel good riding after a meal. Big mistake! I bonked hard on some large hills. I felt lethargic, light-headed, dizzy, and definitely irritable. As soon as I finished, I devoured a turkey sub and a whole Gatorade. I felt much better. Incredible what a little food and drink can do!**
>
> Jessica Truslow, Arlington, MA

believe you are addicted to sugar. This is unlikely. The simple solution is to eat before you get overly hungry. If you crave sweets, you have likely gone too long without eating and have gotten too hungry.

- *Predinner snack attacks*—If you routinely find yourself attacking the package of cookies or box of crackers the minute you get home from work, you are not eating enough during the day. Examine how many calories you need (see chapter 13) and how many you eat during the day. If you eat only 50 percent (or less) of your day's calories by the time you get home from work, you are running a large caloric deficit. The result is extreme hunger and overeating. Eating at least 75 percent of your day's calories before you get home from work should solve this problem.

- *Postdinner grazing*—If you eat dinner, yet you are unsatisfied and nibble or graze all evening long, perhaps, you did not eat enough during the day. Postdinner grazing is usually due to the accumulation of a large caloric deficit created by insufficient eating throughout the day.

What to Eat for Snacks—Snacking does not have to be a hassle. The easier it is, the more likely you are to eat it. You can consume a snack in a matter of a few minutes, the amount of time it takes to eat a yogurt or half a peanut butter sandwich at your desk; a bagel while walking to work; or dried fruit and nuts while riding your bike. The key is to plan for snacks, just as you plan for breakfast, lunch, or dinner and to have foods available. Here are some tips to make snacking easy:

- Choose convenient foods that are not highly perishable and keep them in your car, desk drawer, duffel bag, backpack, briefcase, or handlebar bag.
- If you pack a lunch bag, also pack a snack bag with two snacks' worth of food.
- Pack a larger lunch and save the extra food for your two snacks. For example, make two sandwiches, one for lunch and one to be divided between two snacks.

❝Beef jerky, fresh fruit, yogurt, string cheese, and bagels are the best snacks because they are portable, tasty, low in fat, and easy to find, even at convenience stores. ❞

Kate Riedell, Fairfield, CT

The best sports snacks include wholesome carbohydrates. If you have health-ful snacks on hand, you can avoid the temptations that lurk in every corner store, vending machine, or bakery. Keep a supply of "emergency" food at work, in your bike bag, or car so you are prepared for the afternoon or mid-morning munchies.

Nonperishable snacks to keep in your desk drawer, backpack, or bike bag:
- Cold cereal
- Packets of instant oatmeal
- Pretzels
- Reduced-fat microwave popcorn
- Low-fat whole-grain crackers
- Peanut butter
- Animal crackers
- Graham crackers
- Low-fat granola bars
- Energy bars
- Noodle soups
- Juice boxes
- Dried fruit
- Nuts
- Trail mix

Perishable snacks to keep in the refrigerator at work, portable cooler, or thermal lunch bag:
- Whole-wheat bagels
- English muffins
- Low-fat bran muffins
- Microwaved potato
- Low-fat yogurt
- Thick-crust pizza
- Fresh fruit
- Leftover pasta
- Turkey, tuna, or cheese sandwich
- Low-fat milk or chocolate milk
- Fruit-flavored cottage cheese

- Use the office refrigerator to store a stash of yogurts, cottage cheese, juices, milk, and baby carrots.
- Plan a regular snack time and stick to it. Set the alarm on your computer or watch, if necessary.
- Consider a liquid snack such as low-fat plain or chocolate milk, juice, smoothie, flavored soymilk, or instant hot choco-late made with milk.

Vending-Machine Snacks—Vending-machine cuisine offers tough choices. Choose carefully. You may get lucky and spy healthful options tucked among the candy and chips, such as pretzels, energy bars, fig cookies, juice, yogurt, or even an apple. The good thing about vending-machine snacks is that they are limited in size; if you opt for cookies, you are limited to only four of them instead of the whole bag, and you consume only 200 to 400 calories, not 2,000.

Salads, whether served as a main dish or an accompaniment, are a simple way to boost your intake of vegetables. For the best salad:

- Use fresh or frozen (thawed) vegetables rather than canned.

- Choose a variety of colorful vegetables—dark green lettuce, red tomatoes and peppers, orange carrots—for the most nutrients.

- Monitor the dressing. Don't drown 50 calories of healthful salad ingredients with 400 calories of fatty dressing!

- Consider salad bars at the grocery store. They are an easy and economical alternative to preparing your own.

Here is how some popular salad ingredients compare. Note that the most colorful ones have the most nutritional value.

Salad Ingredient Per 2 cups raw:	Vitamin C (milligrams)	Vitamin A (international units)
Daily Value (recommended intake)	60	5,000
Spinach	50	7,400
Romaine, shredded	20	5,450
Iceberg lettuce, shredded	5	720
Per 1/2 cup raw:		
Carrot slices	5	7,340
Red pepper, chopped	140	2,300
Peas	10	1,480
Tomato, chopped	10	760
Broccoli	40	680
Cucumber slices	0.5	25
Cauliflower	25	5
Mushrooms	1	0

1 cup = 240 millititers
Nutrition information from USDA National Nutrient Database (online)

Outrageous Snacks—If it's an ice cream sundae or other such belt-busting treat that you are craving, it is better to satisfy your hankering by indulging at lunchtime rather than at dinnertime or later. By spending your lunchtime calories on the treat, you can still balance your day's calorie and nutrition budget, and you'll certainly have incentive to train harder that afternoon. You won't destroy your health with this occasional treat as long as your overall diet tends to be wholesome.

For a substantial sports salad that's hearty enough to count as a meal, add extra carbohydrates and protein.

For carbohydrates:
- Dense vegetables, such as sliced sweet potato, peas or corn, or canned beets
- Beans and legumes, such as chickpeas, kidney beans, and three-bean salad
- Tofu or tempeh
- Cooked rice, pasta, bulgur, or couscous
- Fruit: oranges, apples, raisins, grapes, fresh peaches, or mango
- Toasted croutons or bagel chips
- Whole-grain bread or pita bread on the side

For protein:
- Cottage cheese, grated low-fat cheddar, plain yogurt
- Tuna, sardines, diced chicken, or turkey
- Beans and legumes
- Tofu or tempeh
- Boiled egg
- A glass of milk to accompany the salad

For salad dressing:
- Choose from the many low-fat and fat-free bottled salad dressings available in stores and at salad bars.
- If you prefer regular bottled dressings, choose those made with olive oil or canola oil for the health-protective monounsaturated fats.
- To reduce the fat content of regular dressings, dilute them with water or vinegar (for Italian-type dressings), or yogurt or milk (for ranch and other mayonnaise-based dressings).
- If you prefer to use oil and vinegar or if you make your own dressing, use good-quality balsamic or flavored vinegar to reduce or eliminate the need for oil.

- **DINNER**—Dinnertime generally marks the end of the day's work, a time to relax and enjoy a nice meal, that is, if you have the energy to prepare it. The challenge is to arrive at home or at the campground not starving, and with enough energy to prepare a decent, healthy meal. This means eating at least 75 percent of your calories during the day as breakfast, lunch, and snacks.

If you are cooking-challenged, you should know that it is far easier to eat a healthful diet if you know how to cook, even if just a little. You may want to look into basic cooking classes at the local adult education center or community college. A basic, tried-and-true cookbook, such as *Betty Crocker's Cook Book: Everything You Need to Know to Cook Today* (John Wiley & Sons, 2000) can help you learn to cook fast, healthful, and tasty meals. Additionally, touring cyclists might want to pick up a book on camp cooking prior to the tour. But remember, no number of cooking classes or cookbooks will help if you enter the dinner hour too hungry to cook or make wise food choices.

> **For dinners I have a few stand-bys: stirfry, pasta, canned soups, and fajitas, and less frequently, enchiladas, turkey burgers, burritos, and homemade pizza. The bottom line is: it has to be easy, healthy, and fast.**
>
> Tracie Timothy, Salt Lake City, UT

Quick Fixes for Dinner—To make dinner preparation as hassle-free as possible, when at home, you may want to incorporate some of the evening prep work into your morning routine. For example, while you shower or shave for work, you could cook a pot of rice or bake a potato. Use the shopping list on page 22 to keep your kitchen stocked with the fixings for any number of healthful and easy meals. On days you don't want to cook, grocery stores offer convenient ready-to-eat meals, such as hot entrees and side dishes, soup-and-salad bars, deli sandwiches, and rotisserie chicken. These offer a convenient option for touring cyclists who occasionally may not feel like getting out the camp stove.

Rice—Rice is underrated as a sports food. Overshadowed by the more popular dinner starches (like potato and pasta) rice is a rich source of carbohydrates. Preferably you will choose brown rice instead of the refined, white varieties. When you cook rice, make extra. This way, cooked rice is on hand for quick dinner preparation. See *Quick and Easy Rice Ideas* on page 123.

Pasta: A Superfood?—Every biker, regardless of language, understands the word pasta. Pasta parties are universally enjoyed around the world, and many cyclists consider pasta as the preferred food for carbo-loading and recovery. Indeed, many believe pasta to be some kind of superfood, which it is not. Granted, pasta and most other noodles, such as rice, egg, or Chinese noodles, are

● QUICK FIXES FOR DINNER

Here is a list of quick fixes for dinner at home or at campsites when you are touring:

- Pasta with spaghetti sauce plus cooked ground beef or turkey, canned clams, canned beans, tempeh, or tofu
- Canned beans, such as kidney or pinto beans, drained and rinsed and then spooned over rice, pasta, or salad
- Frozen pierogie or burrito served with a side salad
- Potato topped with cooked (frozen) broccoli and cottage cheese, or reheated with black beans, low-fat cheese, and salsa
- English-muffin, flour-tortilla, or pita-bread pizza—top with spaghetti sauce and grated cheese then toast in the oven or toaster oven
- Toasted pita bread filled with hummus or tuna and salad greens
- Bean soup (canned or from the deli) plus fresh fruit and whole-grain bread; chicken soup with added frozen vegetables; vegetable soup with added canned beans
- Large flour tortilla filled with canned refried beans, then topped with low-fat cheese, lettuce, and salsa
- Rotisserie chicken from the grocery store with stuffing and frozen vegetables
- Stirfry made with chicken, tofu, or tempeh, frozen vegetables (or pre washed vegetables from the market or salad bar), your favorite seasonings, and rice
- Baked fish or chicken breast with couscous and fresh fruit
- Pasta salad made with leftover pasta, thawed frozen peas and broccoli, canned tuna or beans, and low-fat salad dressing
- Big salad with lettuce, vegetables, and tofu, kidney beans, boiled egg, deli turkey, or cottage cheese, plus a side of whole-grain bread (see note on salads, page 30)
- Tuna noodle casserole—cream of mushroom soup + cooked noodles + tuna + frozen peas—plus a side salad
- Sandwich—tuna, salmon, or egg salad, toasted cheese and tomato, or peanut butter with raisins—and fresh fruit
- Frozen veggie burger, fish fillet, turkey burger, or lean hamburger on a whole-grain roll with lettuce and tomato
- Omelet with sliced tomato or frozen vegetables and low-fat cheese, and Oven Fries
- For more ideas, see *Quick and Easy Pasta Ideas* on page 119 and *Quick and Easy Rice Ideas* on page 123.

When you cook rice, make extra. Leftover rice can help you prepare a nutritious meal in minutes (If bike touring/camping, use instant rice). For a quick meal and little clean-up we recommend the following:

1. Brown some lean hamburger, ground turkey, tofu, or thin-sliced sliced chicken breast in a large skillet over medium-high heat.

2. Add raw, frozen, or canned vegetables as desired and cook until tender:

   Raw: carrot, onion, celery, peppers, garlic

   Frozen: broccoli, peas, corn, spinach, green beans (these need less time to cook than do raw vegetables)

   Canned: tomatoes or tomato sauce

3. Add the cooked rice and season as desired. Enjoy your healthful, delicious meal.

Here are some good combinations for your rice dish:

- *Mexican:* Beef or chicken + kidney beans + chili powder or taco seasoning + grated reduced-fat cheese + salsa or tomatoes

- *Chinese:* Chicken or tofu + broccoli or frozen mixed vegetables + soy sauce + fresh or powdered ginger

- *Italian:* Turkey sausage + tomato sauce + green beans or peppers + Italian seasoning (basil, thyme, oregano, garlic)

- *All-American:* Ground beef or turkey + onion + canned tomatoes + grated reduced-fat cheese

---

❝For my dinner entree, I eat pasta or rice with beans. A can of beans is so easy to open. I either use the quick cooking rice or make a big batch of rice ahead of time and use it for a couple of days in a row. ❞

MaryAnn Martinez, Concord, MA

carbohydrate-rich, easy to cook, economical, and enjoyed by almost every family member. But in terms of vitamins, minerals, fiber, and protein, plain pasta and noodles are lackluster foods.

Pasta is made from refined or processed flour, wheat that has been stripped of its fiber-rich bran and nutrient-rich germ. With respect to nutrition, plain pasta is really no different than soft white sandwich bread. Whole-wheat pasta, on the other hand, offers more nutrition, most notably fiber. If you don't like the taste or consistency of whole-wheat pasta, try mixing it half and half with traditional pasta.

Don't bank on spinach, tomato, or other such colorful pasta noodles to provide you with much

● SOUP: MMM, MMM GOOD

There are three terrific things about soup. A pot of soup, chili, or stew goes a long way—from fridge or freezer, it makes for many simple, heat-and-eat meals. Soups generally are low in fat and highly nutritious (except for those made with cream or cheese). And a bowl of soup can be a tasty way to consume several servings of vegetables at one meal.

Canned soups and broths are a convenient alternative to homemade, and they can be just as nutritious. However, canned products generally have more sodium than homemade. Individuals on sodium-restricted diets or with high blood pressure should choose low-sodium varieties.

Here are some ways to convert plain ol' canned soup into something special:

- *Combine soups:*
  - Tomato and vegetable
  - Hearty bean or lentil and vegetable
  - Onion or escarole and chicken noodle

- *Add ingredients:*
  - Frozen vegetables: peas, corn, carrots, spinach, or broccoli
  - Fresh chopped parsley, cilantro, or green onion
  - Canned whole or diced tomato
  - Diced, cooked chicken
  - Cooked rice or noodles
  - Frozen tortellini or wontons
  - Canned, drained garbanzo or kidney beans

- *Add seasonings:*
  - Curry powder to chicken soup
  - Cloves to tomato soup
  - Wine, sherry, vermouth to mushroom soup
  - Garlic powder or hot sauce to vegetable soup
  - Cumin and chili powder to bean soup

- *Add toppings:*
  - Parmesan cheese
  - Grated low-fat cheese
  - Toasted bread, cubed
  - Croutons

added nutrition. These contain relatively little actual spinach or tomato, probably a teaspoon or less per cup of cooked pasta, and do not compare nutritionally to a half-cup serving of vegetable eaten with the meal.

The nutritional quality of your pasta meal can go up or down depending on what you add to your pasta. Pasta can be a fat-laden nutritional nightmare if it is smothered with butter, oil, cream sauce, or greasy meat sauces. Or it can be a nutritional superfood if topped with vegetable sauces or lean meat or fish sauces:

Topping	*Nutrients*
• Tomato sauce, canned or homemade	Vitamins A and C, Potassium
• Pesto sauce, made from fresh basil or spinach	Vitamins A and C, Potassium
• Sautéed bell peppers, tomato, and onion	Vitamins A and C, Potassium
• Clam sauce made with a little olive oil	Protein, Zinc, Iron
• Tomato sauce with chicken, lean ground beef or turkey, clams, shrimp, or fish	Protein, Zinc, Iron, Vitamins A and C, Potassium

Pasta and Protein—Pasta is popular not only for carbohydrates but also for being a vegetarian alternative to meat-based meals. However, many cyclists and other athletes live on too much pasta and neglect their protein needs. For example, Joe, an aspiring Olympian, thought his high-carbohydrate, low-fat diet of pasta and tomato sauce seven nights per week was top-notch. He wondered why he felt chronically tired and was not improving despite hard training. The answer was simple. His limited diet was deficient in not only protein but also iron and zinc. He was advised to add a variety of protein-rich choices to his tomato sauce:

• 2 to 3 ounces cooked extra-lean ground beef or turkey
• 1/4 cup grated part-skim mozzarella cheese
• 1/2 cake tofu or tempeh
• 2/3 cup canned, drained kidney or garbanzo beans
• 3 ounces tuna (half of a 6-ounce can)
• 1/2 cup canned clams or shrimp
• 1 cup low-fat cottage cheese

Or, instead of adding protein to the sauce, he would drink two glasses of low-fat milk with the meal. Once he started to supplement the pasta with a variety of proteins, he started to feel better, train and perform better, and recover better.

• **SUMMARY**—If you are like many cyclists who know what they should eat but just don't do it, you need to remember the following keys to a successful sports diet:
• Getting too hungry is probably the biggest problem with most cyclists' diets. Eat appropriately sized meals on a regular

● SPUDS FOR CYCLISTS

Potatoes are pre-wrapped, convenient, nutritious, and rich in carbohydrates, potassium, and vitamin C. A large baked potato offers 65 percent the recommended intake (Daily Value) for vitamin C and all the potassium you'd lose in three hours of sweaty exercise. A sweet potato (or "yam," as it is often mistakenly called) offers the additional health benefits of beta-carotene. Potatoes are a good sports food for meals or snacks. Some cyclists carry baked potatoes in a pocket, as they might a piece of fruit, and munch on them during and after rides when they need an energy booster.

Tips for potatoes:

- Russets are better suited for baking than are the red, white, or gold potatoes, which are preferred for boiling or mashing.
- Store potatoes at room temperature. Refrigerated potatoes quickly become sweet and off-colored.
- Eat the skin (even on sweet potatoes). You'll get more vitamin C and fiber.
- A large, plain restaurant-size baked potato generally has around 200 calories. Be wary of mashed potatoes in a restaurant. They may taste delicious because of the added butter, but they also can add a hundred or more calories of fat to your meal.
- Sweet potatoes can be cooked and eaten in the same manner as other potatoes.

Ideas for baked potatoes:

- Top with a dollop of pesto or spaghetti sauce
- Top with steamed broccoli
- Serve with chili, stew, or bean or lentil soup
- Drizzle with low-fat or fat-free salad dressing
- Top with fat-free sour cream, chopped onion, and grated low-fat cheddar cheese
- Top with low-fat cottage cheese and salsa

- Mash baked sweet potatoes with brown sugar, cinnamon, and orange juice or apple cider
- Make "nachos"—add black beans and grated low-fat cheddar cheese and heat in microwave, then add chopped tomatoes, jalapenos, salsa, and reduced-fat sour cream
- Sprinkle with fresh or dried herbs and seasonings: garlic, basil, thyme, dill, chopped chives
- Enjoy plain with just salsa, ketchup, or mustard

● PASTA, POTATO, OR RICE?

If you have the choice between plain pasta, rice, or potato for dinner, consider the potato. It offers far more vitamin C, potassium, fiber, and overall health value. Here's the lineup for these popular dinner starches:

Food/Amount	Calories	Vitamin C (mg)	Potassium (mg)	Carb. (g)	Fiber (g)
Spaghetti, plain 2 cups cooked (4 ounces dry)	420	0	85	84	4
Spaghetti, 100% whole wheat 2½ cups cooked (4 ounces dry)	420	0	150	84	6
White rice 2 cups cooked (½ cup dry)	410	0	110	88	1
Brown rice 2 cups cooked (½ cup dry)	430	0	165	88	7
Potato, baked, with skin 2 medium	320	30	1,850	72	8
Sweet potato, baked, with skin 2 medium	200	45	1,080	46	8

2 cups = 480 milliliters; 4 ounces = 112 grams
Nutrition information from food labels, USDA National Nutrient Database (online), and J. Pennington, 2004, Bowes & Church's Food Values of Portions Commonly Used, 18th ed. (Philadelphia: Lippincott, Williams & Wilkins)

schedule to prevent yourself from getting too hungry. Notice how your diet deteriorates when you get too hungry.

- Plan ahead for meals and snacks. Have healthy, convenient foods available. Go grocery shopping regularly and keep your kitchen stocked.
- Spend your calories on a variety of wholesome foods. Target three food groups per meal; two per snack.
- Hearty carbohydrate-based meals are the foundation of an active cyclist's sports diet.
- Nutritious meals need not be a burden to prepare and can be made in a matter of minutes.

CHAPTER 4

Vitamins, Minerals, and Other Dietary Supplements

VITAMINS AND OTHER DIETARY SUPPLEMENTS ARE GROWING IN POPU-
larity. Surveys suggest that 75 percent to 90 percent of athletes take some type of supplement with hopes it will stave off illness, enhance performance, and make them healthy. The Food
and Drug Administration loosely regulates dietary supplements.
Because the FDA does not require the stringent pre-market review
that it requires for drugs and food additives, dietary supplements
can go to market and be advertised with little data proving their
effectiveness or guaranteeing their safety.

Vitamins and minerals have been for many
years the subjects of large research studies on
health and disease. It is well-established that
deficiencies in these essential nutrients cause
disease and that supplementing with a food
source or pill reverses, prevents, or attenuates
the disease. Other dietary supplements, such as
herbs, amino acids, phytochemicals, on the
other hand, have not been as widely studied,
and there is little data to prove their usefulness
in health or athletic performance.

Let's take a look at some of what is and is
not known about dietary supplements, and then
you can decide your path towards optimal nutrition.

> **I have always believed eating right is the best way to get all nutrients. With my caloric intake and the variety of foods I eat, I should be fine.**
>
> Ed Kross, Framingham, MA

● **VITAMINS AND MINERALS**—Vitamins and minerals are essential nutrients that your body cannot make. They perform
important jobs in your body. For example, thiamin (a B-vita-

min) helps to convert glucose into energy; iron transports oxygen to your muscles; and calcium and vitamin D are used to make and maintain bone cells.

Are You Getting Enough?—You do not need to take a supplement pill to meet your vitamin and mineral needs. You can get the recommended intake of these nutrients by eating a variety of wholesome foods from the food pyramid. Most athletes consume more than enough nutrients simply by virtue of their high calorie intake. A hungry cyclist needs more calories, eats more food, and therefore gets more nutrients than someone who is less active and eats less. Plus, many of the foods that cyclists eat are highly fortified with extra vitamins and minerals, breakfast cereals and energy bars in particular. A serving of cereal may contain a full day's supply of many vitamins and minerals. If you think you are not getting enough vitamins and minerals, first take a look at your diet to see if you are eating a variety of foods from all the food groups in the pyramid (see chapter 1). Then take a look at the nutrients in the fortified foods you eat. If you eat a well-balanced diet that includes fortified foods, you likely are getting more than enough vitamins and minerals without taking a supplement.

People Who Should Take a Supplement—Some situations put you at risk for nutritional deficiencies, such as:

- *Restricting calories.* Eating fewer calories = eating fewer foods = consuming fewer nutrients.
- *Eating a repetitive diet of bagels and pasta.* A steady diet of bagels, bread, and pasta may leave you lacking in the nutrients found in other food groups, such as iron and zinc (from meat), vitamins A and C (from fruits and vegetables), and calcium and vitamin D (from milk).
- *Skimping on fruits and vegetables.* A diet lacking fruits and vegetables is likely lacking in vitamins C and A, fiber, and antioxidants.
- *Lactose intolerance or avoidance of dairy foods.* Avoidance of dairy foods can lead to a diet deficient in calcium, vitamin D, and riboflavin.
- *Over-indulging in fats and sweets.* Filling up on nutrient-poor foods like candy and chips leaves you less hungry for healthful foods.
- *Pregnant or contemplating pregnancy.* Women require additional nutrients before and during pregnancy to help prevent birth defects. All women who may become pregnant are advised to take a multivitamin with 400 micrograms of folacin (folic acid, a B-vitamin) to help prevent brain damage in the fetus. Women who are expecting should check with their physicians about which supplements they need to take.
- *Vegetarian.* People who abstain from animal products are at risk for developing B12, iron, vitamin D, iron, zinc, and protein deficiencies. This risk can be reduced or eliminated by choosing a well-balanced vegetarian diet.
- *Illness.* People who are sick may eat fewer calories and thus fewer nutrients, putting them at risk for deficiencies.
- *Being a senior.* Seniors may require fewer calories and eat less than younger, more active adults, so they may not get all the nutrients they need.

If any of these situations applies to you, be sure to make dietary changes to get more of the nutrients you need and consider taking a multivitamin and mineral pill.

Many athletes wonder if exercise increases their requirement for vitamins and minerals. The answer is no. There are no studies to date that have documented a physiological need for extra doses of vitamins or minerals for athletes. Nor is there evidence that vitamin and mineral supplementation improves performance, despite supplement industry claims. Extra vitamins and minerals do not increase muscle mass or strength, enhance endurance, or offer a competitive edge in athletes who are adequately nourished.

Some people, even those who eat well, take a supplement as health insurance. Many believe it to be a magic bullet that will potentially make them healthier, prevent or cure disease, or help them to live longer. While taking a simple, one-a-day multivitamin and mineral pill will certainly not hurt you, it remains to be seen if taking doses beyond the RDA (Recommended Dietary Allowance) will improve your health if you already eat a good diet and have no nutritional deficiencies.

Food Offers More Than Pills—Plant foods contain hundreds, perhaps thousands, of compounds called phytochemicals that provide protection against disease. Researchers continue to investigate whether consuming extra phytochemicals, for example lycopene, leutein, and carotenoids, in the form of supplements will reduce the incidence of cancer and heart disease. So far, the results are disappointing.

❝I prefer to get my vitamins and minerals from foods, but just to make sure I am not missing anything, I take a multivitamin. ❞

MaryAnn Martinez, Concord, MA

If you choose to take a vitamin and mineral supplement, remember that while a supplement pill may stave off major nutrient deficiencies, no amount of any supplement will compensate for a lousy, hit-or-miss diet and stress-filled lifestyle. We highly recommend that you make the effort to eat your nutrients through food and only turn to supplements in special circumstances such as those listed previously.

● **SPORTS SUPPLEMENTS**—Some cyclists look beyond simple vitamins and minerals to sports supplements hoping to increase their energy, stamina, and muscle mass, and improve their athletic performance. Many sports foods, gels, or beverages are fortified with antioxidant vitamins, mega-doses of B-vitamins, herbs, caffeine, and other compounds and claim to enhance athletic performance. Will these substances really give you a competitive edge? The odds are no.

Because the FDA poorly regulates dietary supplements for quality, purity, or effectiveness, you can't be quite sure what or how much of a substance you are getting, or if (or how) it will affect you. Also consider that the sports food industry is growing by leaps and bounds, and a plethora of products is widely available. With such competition, companies are adding everything from ginseng to branched-chain amino acids to their energy bars, gels, and drinks claiming it will boost performance or enhance immunity. In actuality, there is scanty scientific evidence showing these substances are helpful at all.

Below are some of the supplements of interest to many cyclists with information to help you make the appropriate decision.

Caffeine—Many cyclists routinely drink a cup of coffee before they head out, saying it clears the mental cobwebs, energizes them, and helps them to work harder. Caffeine's energy-enhancing effect is likely due to its ability to make exercise seem easier. Caffeine stimulates the brain and may delay the perception of fatigue, allowing you to work harder for longer. Once thought to have a dehydrating effect, current research indicates caffeine is not dehydrating in athletes accustomed to consuming caffeinated beverages (Armstrong 2002).

If you do not ordinarily consume caffeine, you'll feel a greater buzz than someone who consumes it regularly. Too much caffeine may cause the jitters, probably the last thing you want when faced with a challenging ride or event. If you are looking to caffeine to make you feel less tired or more awake, you may want to ask yourself if you are getting enough sleep, overtraining, or stressed. Perhaps the most justifiable reason for consuming caffeine is to promote a pre-ride bowel movement!

B-Vitamins—Thiamin, Niacin, B6, Riboflavin, B12, pantothenic acid, biotin, and folate are referred to as B-complex vitamins. B-vitamins are essential in all metabolic and energy-producing processes in your body, and the need for B increases with intense exercise. This has led to the assumption that B supplementation will enhance energy and improve athletic performance. Scientific research does not support this assumption (Webster et al. 1997, Schwenk and Costley 2002).

A hungry cyclist is likely to eat more than enough B-vitamins to meet his or her requirements. Most sports supplements, foods, and drinks contain several or all of these vitamins. Grain foods such as breakfast cereals, breads, and pasta are often enriched or fortified, and B is found naturally in a wide variety of foods.

Food Sources for Selected B Vitamins:

Thiamin (B1)	pork; whole grains; enriched cereal, rice, corn tortillas
Niacin (B3)	turkey, chicken, tuna, beef, peanuts, legumes, enriched cereal and pasta
Pyridoxine (B6)	chicken, pork, fish, whole grains, legumes
Riboflavin	milk, yogurt, eggs, whole-grain bread, enriched grain products
B12	primarily animal foods: meat, milk, chicken, fish
Folate	fortified breakfast cereals, rice, pasta, and bread; orange juice, lentils, legumes, spinach, broccoli, peanuts
Pantothenic acid	meat, poultry, fish, whole grains, legumes, yogurt, milk
Biotin	egg, whole grains, wheat germ, pancakes

Beta-carotene, Vitamins C and E, Selenium—These compounds act as antioxidants. They deactivate destructive free radicals, compounds in the body that contribute to health problems such as heart disease and cancer. The bulk of scientific studies conclude that taking antioxidant supplements does not reduce your risk for disease. Supplementing with vitamin C, or C and E before a strenuous distance will also not reduce oxidative or immune changes (Nieman et al. 2002) or reduce muscle damage (Dawson et al. 2002). The body can handle the physical stress of intense exercise without the use of supplements. Your best bet it to eat a diet naturally rich in these nutrients—abundant fruits and vegetables. See page 46 for foods rich in antioxidants.

Creatine—Creatine is a naturally occurring compound found in meat and fish. Muscles use creatine phosphate to generate energy for one to ten seconds of intense work (such as in sprinting or weightlifting). In people who respond to creatine supplements, muscles may perform better during these brief, all-out exercise bouts (Terjung et al. 2000). By being able to work harder, the muscles can become bigger. But not everyone responds to creatine (Kilduff et al. 2002). The research to date suggests no physical harm from creatine if it is taken in the recommended doses. But as with all dietary supplements, creatine is not regulated for quality and what you buy may not be what you get.

Glycerol—Glycerol retains fluid in the body. Glycerol (or glycerate) may be added to commercial sports fluid supplements and gels claiming to "enhance sport performance." Exercise scientists are conducting research to determine if glycerol can help healthy athletes maintain hydration and improve exercise performance. So far, evidence is conflicting. While glycerol supplementation improves hydration status, it may or may not improve athletic performance (Magal et al. 2003, Montner et al. 1996, Wagner 1999). Side effects may include headache and blurred vision, which could interfere with performance and present a safety hazard. For more information on hydration see chapter 7.

Ginseng—Ginseng is a plant that has been used medicinally for thousands of years in China, Japan, and Korea. Some believe that ginseng boosts mood and energy, decreases cardiovascular disease, improves athletic performance, and even acts as an aphrodisiac. These claims have yet to be supported scientifically. Most of the studies on ginseng have been poorly controlled, offer conflicting results and are difficult to interpret. There are no good studies that support the use of ginseng for any purpose, including improving or enhancing athletic performance (Bahrke et al. 2000, Engels et al. 1997).

Protein, Amino Acids, and Branched-chain Amino Acids—All protein, whether in foods you eat or in your muscles, is made up of amino acids, the building blocks of protein. There are 21 amino acids. Your body can manufacture all but nine of the amino acids. These are referred to as "essential" amino acids because you must consume them in your diet. When you eat protein-rich foods, your body breaks down the protein into amino acids. The amino acids circulate through the blood and if needed, they are recombined to build various tissues in the body. If you overeat protein, the extra amino acids are burned for energy or stored as fat.

Until science proves otherwise, your best bet for getting beta-carotene, vitamin C, and other antioxidants important for good health is to eat foods that are naturally rich in these nutrients. Use this list to guide you to an appropriate (and natural) intake of several of these health-protective nutrients.

Vitamin C: Daily Value (DV)* = 60 milligrams (mg)
The best sources include fruits (especially citrus) and vegetables.

Food	Amount	Vitamin C (mg)	%DV
Kiwi	1	75	125
Orange	1	80	135
Grapefruit juice	1 cup	80	135
Cantaloupe	1/4 melon	70	120
Broccoli, cooked	1 cup	20	200

Vitamin E: Daily Value = 30 international units (IU)
The best sources are plant oils like vegetable oils and nuts. Be sure to include some of these healthful, high-fat foods in your daily calorie budget.

Food	Amount	Vitamin E (IU)	%DV
Sunflower seeds	1/4 cup	12	40
Almonds	1/4 cup	12	40
Wheat germ	1/4 cup	7	23
Safflower oil	1 tablespoon	4.5	15
Peanut butter	2 tablespoons	4.5	15

Beta-carotene
Bright orange and yellow fruits and vegetables and dark green vegetables are rich sources of beta-carotene and other health-protective carotenoids. Beta-carotene is converted to vitamin A in the body and it is expressed as "vitamin A" on food labels. The Daily Value for vitamin A is 5,000 international units (IU).

Food	Amount	Vitamin A (IU)	%DV
Sweet potato, baked	1 medium	21,900	440
Carrot, raw	1 medium	20,250	410
Spinach, cooked	1/2 cup	7,400	150
Mango	1	6,420	130
Cantaloupe	1 cup	5,160	100
Butternut/buttercup squash, boiled, mashed	1/2 cup	4,000	80
Romaine lettuce, shredded	1 cup	2,730	55
Broccoli, cooked	1/2 cup	1,530	30

1 cup = 240 milliliters; 1 tablespoon = 15 milliliters; 3 ounces = 85 grams

Selenium: Daily Value = 55 micrograms (mcg)
The best sources for selenium generally are nuts, meats, seafood, and poultry. Foods vary greatly in their selenium content depending on where the food was grown. Selenium is toxic in high doses. Eating a wide variety of foods is your best bet in getting enough (and not too much) selenium.

Food	Amount	Selenium (mcg)	%DV
Sunflower seeds	¹/₄ cup	25	45
Tuna, canned, drained	3 ounces	65	95
Shrimp, cooked	3 ounces	35	60
Chicken breast, skinless, roasted	3 ounces	20	35
Beef, lean, ground, broiled	3 ounces	20	30
Egg	1 large	15	20

Nutrition information from food labels; USDA National Nutrient Database online at www.nal.usda.gov/fnic/foodcomp/; J. Pennington, 2004, Bowes & Church's Food Values of Portions Commonly Used, 18th ed. (Philadelphia: Lippincott, Williams & Wilkins); and the Office of Dietary Supplements (USDA) online at http://ods.od.nih.gov

^The Daily Value is the amount of a nutrient that meets the needs of most adults and is based on a 2,000-calorie diet.

Some cyclists wonder if taking extra amino acids will help their performance or enhance immunity. To date, no scientific evidence indicates that individual amino acids have a body-building, performance-enhancing, or immune-stimulating effect. Taking a protein supplement on top of an adequate diet (0.5 gram of protein per pound of body weight, or 1.0 gram per kilogram) will not enhance muscle strength or size (Godard, Williamson et al. 2002).

Three of the essential amino acids are branched-chain amino acids (BCAA) and include isoleucine, leucine, and valine. These have been studied for their possible role in delaying fatigue during exercise, in part because BCAA levels decline with exercise. To date, the studies are inconclusive. Some show improved mental function or reductions in perceived exertion with supplementation of BCAA, but most do not demonstrate a positive effect on performance (Fragakis 2003). You should know that consuming carbohydrates before, during, and after exercise prevents the decline of BCAA during exercise and is proven to enhance performance (Davis 1995).

The amino acids in supplements are not better than the amino acids (as protein) found in food naturally. You can easily get all the essential amino acids you need by eating regular food and getting adequate protein. The advantages of food include more vitamins, minerals, and other nutrients. Plus, food costs much less than supplements: A 6-ounce can of tuna costs $0.99 and provides 30 grams of protein; a PowerBar ProteinPlus costs $1.95 and provides 24 grams of protein. Until more research proves otherwise, your best bet for maximum performance is to get your amino acids by eating protein-rich foods such as chicken, meat, fish, soy, and dairy products as part of your healthy diet. See chapter 5 for more on protein.

• AM I SICK, OR JUST TIRED? DO I NEED A SUPPLEMENT?—

Exercise energizes many people, enhances their productivity, and relieves their stress. But some cyclists complain of chronic fatigue. They feel run-down, dragged-out, and overwhelmingly exhausted. If this sounds familiar, you may wonder if a vitamin pill or other dietary supplement would solve the problem.

Perhaps you can relate to Jim, a 43-year-old long-distance cyclist. A busy single professional, he bemoaned, "My diet is awful. I rarely eat fruits or vegetables. I live on fast foods. What vitamins should I take?" Jim lived alone and hated to cook for just himself. He rarely ate breakfast, barely ate lunch, but always collapsed after a long day with a generous fast-food feast. He struggled to wake up in the morning, stay awake during afternoon meetings, and grind through his training rides and gym workouts. Jim hoped some vitamins pills would restore his energy. Doubtful.

Nancy evaluated Jim's diet, calculated that he had 3,000 calories in his daily energy budget (1,000 calories per section of the day, i.e. morning, midday, evening), and suggested a few simple food changes that could result in higher energy, greater stamina, and better biking. Nancy explored the following questions looking for solutions to Jim's fatigue. Perhaps the answers will offer solutions for your energy problems, if you have similar concerns.

• *Are you tired due to low blood sugar?* Jim skipped not only breakfast but also missed lunch because he didn't have time. He would doze off in the afternoon because he had low blood sugar. With little glucose to feed his brain, he ended up feeling sleepy. The solution was to choose to make time to eat. Just as he chose to sleep later in the morning, he could choose to get up five minutes earlier for breakfast. He could also choose to stop working for five or ten minutes to eat lunch.

- *Is your diet too low in carbohydrates?* Jim's fast but fatty food choices filled his stomach, but left his muscles poorly fueled with inadequate glycogen to support his training program. Higher-carbohydrate snacks and meals would fuel his muscles and help maintain a higher blood sugar level. He'd have energy for mental work as well as physical exercise.
- *Are you iron-deficient and anemic?* Jim ate little red meat and consequently little iron, an important mineral in red blood cells that helps carry oxygen to exercising muscles. Iron-deficiency anemia can result in needless fatigue during exercise. Jim was taught how to boost his dietary iron intake, with or without meat (see chapter 5). He was referred for blood tests (hemoglobin, hematocrit, ferritin, serum iron, and total iron-binding capacity) to rule out anemia.
- *Are you getting enough sleep?* Jim's complaint about being chronically tired was justified because he was tired both mentally (from his intense job) and physically (from his strenuous training). He worked from 8 a.m. to 8 p.m. If he didn't ride at lunchtime, he'd ride or head to the gym after work. By the time he got home, ate dinner, and unwound, midnight had rolled around. The wake-up bell at 6:30 a.m came all too soon, especially since he often had trouble falling asleep due to having eaten such a large dinner. Nancy encouraged Jim to try to get more sleep by eating lighter dinners, such as soup and a sandwich, or cereal. He could accomplish this by eating a bigger breakfast and eating his main meal at lunch (lower-fat Chinese meals, pizza, pasta). By trading in 1,200 of his evening calories for 600 more calories at breakfast and 600 more calories at lunch, he could spend less time preparing and eating dinner at night. He could eat less and hopefully get to sleep earlier and with a less-full stomach.
- *Are you overtraining?* Jim took pride in the fact that he had not missed a day of training in three years, yet he felt discouraged he wasn't improving despite harder training. Nancy

questioned whether he was a compulsive exerciser who pun-ished his body or a serious cyclist who trained wisely and took rest days. One or two rest days or easy days per week are an essential part of a training program; they allow the body to replenish its depleted muscle glycogen.

- *Are you stressed or depressed?* Jim not only had a stressful job but was also dealing with the stress and depression associated with family problems, to say nothing of the challenges of train-ing. Since he was feeling a bit helpless with this situation, Nancy encouraged him to successfully control and take pride in at least one aspect of his life: his diet. Simple dietary improvements would help him feel physically and mentally better about him-self. This would be very energizing in itself.

If you can answer 'yes' to many of the questions above, you may be able to resolve your fatigue with better eating, sleeping, and training habits, not with supplements. Simply experiment with the food suggestions in this book and you will transform your current low-energy patterns into a food plan for success.

- **SUMMARY**—Most cyclists can consume all the vitamins and minerals and other nutrients needed for good health by eating a variety of foods from the all of the food groups.
- Extra vitamins and minerals do not enhance performance, increase energy, improve strength and endurance, or lend a competitive edge if you are already adequately nourished and suffer no nutritional deficiencies.
- By eating hearty and healthful cyclist's portions on a regular schedule throughout the day, you'll consume the vitamins, minerals, and calories you need to fight fatigue and support your exercise program.
- Protein supplements on top of an adequate diet will not improve muscle strength or size.
- Remember that dietary and sports supplements are not well-studied, are not regulated for purity and dosage, lack scien-tific evidence to prove their effectiveness, and most likely will not improve your athletic performance.
- If you want more information about supplements, here are two online sources:
  www.nlm.nih.gov/medlineplus/herbalmedicine.html
  www.dietary-supplements.info.nih.gov

CHAPTER 5

Protein for Cyclists

OME CYCLISTS BELIEVE IF THEY EAT A LOT OF PROTEIN, THEY WILL build a lot of muscle. Too bad this isn't the case. If it were true, we could simply devour large portions of meat and end up like Lance Armstrong or Greg Lemond! Other cyclists ignore protein and may be at risk for protein deficiency, for example, vegetarians who don't eat enough beans or touring cyclists eat too much oatmeal and pasta, but not enough peanut butter.

When you are selecting your sports diet, be sure to include the right balance of protein. Ten percent to 15 percent of your calories should come from protein. This relatively small amount of protein is needed to build and repair muscles, maintain your immune system, and make red blood cells, enzymes, and hormones. Eating excess protein offers no benefits to a sports diet. The extra protein you eat does not turn into extra muscle; it is either burned for energy or stored as fat. What does build muscles is resistance exercise—in the form of lifting weights or pushing hard on pedals when you are grinding up a steep hill—accompanied by a healthful

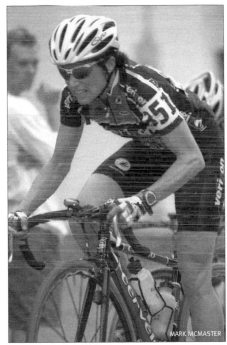

To get to the finish line, you need adequate protein as well as abundant carbohydrates.

MARK MCMASTER

sports diet. Fueling your muscles with wholesome carbohydrates, not excessive amounts of protein, assures you will have the energy to perform muscle-building exercise. Eating too little protein leads to chronic fatigue, anemia, lack of athletic improvement, muscle wasting, and an overall run-down feeling. Iron (prevents anemia) and zinc (helps with healing) deficiencies can occur with a protein-poor diet, since they are primarily found in protein-rich foods.

● **HOW MUCH IS ENOUGH?**—The current Recommended Dietary Allowance for protein is 0.4 grams of protein per pound (0.8 grams per kilogram) of body weight per day for most healthy, sedentary adults. Cyclists in training need more, approximately 0.5 to 0.9 grams of protein per pound (1.0 to 2.0 grams per kilogram). That's about 65 to 125 grams of protein each day for a cyclist weighing 140 pounds (63 kilograms); 80 to 160 grams of protein for someone weighing 180 pounds (82 kilograms). Growing teenagers, athletes building new muscles, long-distance cyclists, and dieters restricting calories should target the higher end of the protein range. On calorie-restricted diets, protein is burned for fuel and is not used for muscle repair and maintenance.

In order to meet your protein needs, each meal should consist of a foundation of grains (including whole grains), fruit, and vegetables. A serving of protein-rich food should be included as an accompaniment to each meal. The following menu gives an example of foods you could eat to get approximately 100 grams of protein in a day, enough for a 180-pound cyclist. Keep in mind that most grains and starchy vegetables provide protein, usually two to three grams per serving.

- *Breakfast:* 8 ounces low-fat milk (8 grams protein) on cereal
- *Snack:* 2 tablespoons peanut butter (8 grams protein) on bread
- *Lunch:* 4 ounces turkey and 1 slice of cheese (30 + 6 grams protein) in a sandwich
- *Snack:* 8 ounces low-fat yogurt (8 grams protein)
- *Dinner:* 4 ounces meatballs (30 grams protein) with pasta and 1/2 cup kidney beans (7 grams protein) on a salad

● **VEGETARIANS AND PROTEIN**—It is possible for vegetarians to consume enough protein to build muscles and maintain health if

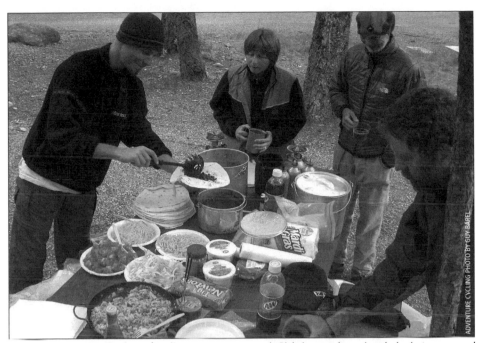

Touring cyclists prepare bean burritos at a campground. Rich in protein and carbohydrates, canned beans are a convenient alternative to meat or poultry.

they choose their diets carefully. The key is to eat plenty of high-protein foods that contain a variety of the essential amino acids, the building blocks your body requires for making and maintaining muscle. Animal sources of protein—meat, fish, poultry, eggs, and milk—offer complete protein, that is, they contain a good balance of all of the essential amino acids. Plant proteins, such as grains, nuts, and legumes, have limited amounts of some of these amino acids. Someone who eats no animal proteins (a vegan) must therefore eat a variety of plant proteins to get sufficient amounts of the essential amino acids. It is not necessary to combine proteins meal-by-meal (for example, rice with beans); just be sure to eat enough protein-rich foods over the course of the day.

● **RED MEAT: EAT OR AVOID...?**—Red meats such as beef, pork, veal, and lamb present a dilemma for many cyclists. Meat is an excellent source of protein. It is rich in iron and zinc, two minerals necessary for optimal health and athletic performance. On the other hand, meat contributes saturated fat and cholesterol to the diet, and it present ethical and environmental issues for

If you wonder if you are eating the right amount of protein, you can estimate your daily protein needs by multiplying your weight by 0.5 to 0.9 grams of protein per pound (1.1 to 2.0 grams of protein per kilogram).

Daily Protein Requirements

	Grams of protein per pound of body weight	Grams of protein if you weigh:		
		120 lb	150 lb	180 lb
RDA for sedentary adult	0.4	50	60	70
Recreational cyclist, adult	0.5-0.7	60-85	75-105	90-125
Endurance cyclist, adult	0.6-0.7	70-85	90-105	110-125
Growing teenage athlete	0.7-0.9	85-110	105-135	125-160
Cyclist building muscle mass	0.7-0.8	85-95	105-120	125-145
Cyclist restricting calories	0.8-0.9	95-110	120-135	145-160
Maximum requirement for adults	0.9	110	135	160

Use food labels and the following chart to calculate your protein intake. Pay close attention to portion sizes!

Protein Content of Some Commonly Eaten Foods

Food	Protein (grams)
Tuna, 1 can (6.5 ounces)	40
Chicken or turkey breast, roasted 4 ounces	35
Beef, pork, cooked, 4 ounces	30
Salmon, cooked, 4 ounces	30
Egg, 1 large	7
Egg white, from 1 large egg	3
Soynuts, ¼ cup roasted	16
Tofu, raw, firm, ½ cup cubes	10
Peanut butter, 2 tablespoons	8
Black beans, ½ cup	7
Soymilk, 1 cup	5-7
Hummus, ½ cup	6
Almonds, 1 ounce (24 nuts)	6
Cottage cheese, ½ cup	14
Milk, 1 cup	8-10
Cheddar cheese, 1 ounce	8
Yogurt, 1 cup	8-10

Food	Protein (grams)
Pasta, 2 ounces dry, or 1 cup cooked	8
Oatmeal, ½ cup dry, or 1 cup cooked	6
Rice, 1/3 cup dry, or 1 cup cooked	4
Cold cereal, 1 ounce	2-3
Bread, 1 slice	2
Potato, white or sweet, 1 small, baked w/skin	2-3
Peas, ½ cup cooked	4

Fruits, watery vegetables
Most fruits and vegetables have negligible amounts of protein. They may contribute a total of five to ten grams of protein per day, depending on how much of them you eat.

Nutrition information from food labels, USDA National Nutrient Database (online), and J. Pennington, 2004, Bowes & Church's Food Values of Portions Commonly Used, 18th ed. (Philadelphia: Lippincott, Williams & Wilkins)

1 cup = 240 milliliters;
1 tablespoon = 15 milliliters; 1 ounce = 28 grams

some individuals. Whether you choose to eat meat or not, you can get all the nutrients needed to support your cycling and promote good health. If you eat red meat, select lean cuts of meat and eat them in moderation. If you avoid meat, take care to eat wisely and include plenty of other protein-rich sources. To eat or not eat meat is a personal decision to which there is no right or wrong answer. Here are some nutrition facts to help you decide if including a small amount of red meat in your weekly menu may enhance the quality of your diet.

Meat vs. Plant Protein—Animal protein adds up quickly. Four ounces (112 grams) of cooked red meat, chicken, or fish is roughly the size of a deck of playing cards and has 25 to 30 grams of protein. Plant proteins can provide a lot of protein too, if you eat enough of them. If you eat only a little peanut butter (2 tablespoons = 9 grams of protein) on a lunchtime sandwich and just a sprinkling of garbanzo beans (1/2 cup = 7 grams protein) on a dinnertime salad, you will fall short of meeting your protein needs. Unlike meat proteins, plant proteins offer the benefit of fiber and health-protective phytochemicals. For more on protein in foods, see *How to Balance Your Protein Intake* on page 54.

> **" I've been a vegetarian for 15 years. Every morning, I put a scoop of soy granules on my whole-grain cereal, top it with soymilk, and enjoy it for a protein-rich start to my day. I consume a ton of fresh veggies, fruit, whole grains, beans, and tofu everyday, with an almost puritanical effort to make every calorie be worthwhile. "**
>
> Charles Breer, St. Paul, MN

Meat, Cholesterol, and Fat—Animals and all food products derived from them contain cholesterol. Plants do not. Even the leanest meats, seafood, and low-fat milk contain some cholesterol. People often mistakenly associate cholesterol content of food with fat content. That perception holds true for red meat (it can be both high in fat and high in cholesterol), but it is not true for all foods. For example, peanut butter is a high-fat food that is cholesterol-free; shrimp is a very low-fat food that is cholesterol-rich. Fat and cholesterol therefore should be regarded separately.

Generally speaking, most animal proteins have similar cholesterol values: 70 to 80 milligrams of cholesterol per four-ounce

● BEANS

- Beans are not only a good source of protein but also carbohydrates, B-vitamins (such as folic acid), and fiber. When added to an overall low-fat diet, they may help lower elevated blood cholesterol levels.
- If beans cause you intestinal problems, eat smaller amounts. If you cook your own beans, be sure to soak them long enough (and discard the water) before cooking. You can also try Beano, a product that when added to beans helps reduce gas formation.

Bean ideas:

- Sauté garlic and onions in a little oil; add canned, drained beans; add chopped fresh tomato; and enjoy it warm or cold.
- Add canned, drained beans to salads, pasta, soups, and stews.
- Make your own bean dip: Puree canned, drained black or pinto beans, a dash of chili powder, cumin, garlic, and/or salsa in a food processor (add water as needed). Use as a cold vegetable dip. Or, top with cheese, heat in the microwave, and use as a topping for a baked potato or as a filling for a burrito.
- Try varieties of hummus that are commercially available, such as roasted pepper hummus, garlic-lover's, and black olive. Spread on (preferably whole-wheat) lavash, pita bread, or flour tortilla, add some crisp vegetables, and roll it up for a "walkabout" sandwich.

> **❝I tend to eat vegan in my daily diet for personal reasons but have learned over the years to listen to my body and if on occasion I really crave steak, well, I have it. ❞**
>
> MaryAnn Martinez, Concord, MA

serving. The American Heart Association recommends that healthy people with normal blood cholesterol levels consume less than 300 milligrams of cholesterol per day. Small portions of red meat can certainly fit those requirements.

In terms of heart health, the cholesterol content of meat is of less concern than the saturated fat content. Fatty meats such as greasy hamburgers, pepperoni, juicy steaks, and sausage are poor choices. Lean meats, such as London broil, extra-lean ground beef, top-round roast beef, lean ham, and pork loin, provide less saturated fat and are better choices for a healthy sports diet. See chapter 6 for more information on fat and cholesterol.

Meat and Iron—Failure to consume adequate iron can lead to anemia, a chronic depletion of iron-rich red blood cells that will leave you weak, tired, vulnerable to illness, and unable to

Here a few ideas to help you with a meat-free diet that has adequate protein.

Breakfast:
- Cold cereal (preferably iron-enriched, as noted on the label): Add milk, yogurt, or soymilk, and sprinkle with a few nuts.
- Oatmeal, oat bran, and other hot cereals: Add peanut butter, almonds or other nuts, and/or powdered milk.
- Toast, bagels: Top with low-fat cheese, cottage cheese, or peanut butter.

Snacks:
- Assorted nuts
- Peanut butter on rice cakes or crackers
- Yogurt (Note: Frozen yogurt has only 4 grams of protein per cup, as compared to 8 grams of protein per cup of regular yogurt.)

Lunch and Dinner:
- *Salads:* Add tofu, tempeh, chickpeas, three-bean salad, marinated kidney beans, low-fat cottage cheese, sunflower seeds, chopped nuts.
- *Protein-rich salad dressing:* Add salad seasonings to plain yogurt, or blenderized tofu or cottage cheese (diluted with milk or yogurt).
- *Spaghetti sauce:* Add diced tofu, or canned, drained kidney beans.
- *Pasta:* Choose protein-enriched pastas that offer 13 grams of protein per cup (as compared to 8 grams per cup of regular pasta). Top with grated part-skim mozzarella cheese.
- *Potato:* Bake or microwave, then top with canned beans, baked beans, or low-fat cottage cheese.
- *Hearty soups:* Choose lentil, split pea, bean, and minestrone.
- *Hummus:* Try hummus with pita or tortillas.
- *Cheese pizza:* Half of a 12-inch pizza has about 40 grams of protein.
- *Burrito:* Top a flour or corn tortilla with canned refried beans and low-fat cheese.
- *Vegetarian burgers and dogs:* Try a soy "hamburger" patty or "hotdog" on a whole-grain bun.

perform at your best. Red meat is arguably one of the best dietary sources of iron for two reasons. First, red meat contains more iron per ounce than fish or poultry. Second, the iron in animal protein, known as heme-iron, is absorbed more easily than the iron from plant sources. If you eat an iron-poor diet and are tempted to simply take an iron supplement, note that animal iron is better absorbed than the iron in a pill.

● CHICKEN AGAIN?

If you are tired of boring baked chicken breast, spice it up with one of these ideas. Remove and discard the skin before preparing.

- Spread with Dijon mustard and sprinkle with Parmesan cheese
- Spread with honey and sprinkle with curry powder
- Marinate for an hour or overnight in Italian dressing
- Spread with honey mustard, bottled barbeque sauce, or bottled Asian stir-fry sauce
- Dip in milk or plain yogurt and roll in cracker crumbs, crumbled stuffing mix, or flavored bread crumbs

Place in baking pan lined with foil (for easy clean up) and bake uncovered at 350°F (175°C) for 20 to 30 minutes or until done.

● HOW TO BOOST YOUR IRON INTAKE

- The recommended intake for iron is 8 milligrams for men and 18 milligrams for women per day. Women have higher iron needs to replace the iron lost from menstrual bleeding. Women who are post-menopausal require only 8 milligrams of iron per day.
- Iron from animal products is absorbed better than that from plant products.
- A source of vitamin C at each meal enhances iron absorption.

Animal Sources (best absorbed)	Iron (mg)	Vegetables	Iron (mg)
		Spinach, ½ cup cooked	3
Beef liver, 4 ounces, cooked	7	Broccoli, ½ cup cooked	1
Beef, 4 ounces, cooked	3	**Beans**	
Shrimp, 4 ounces, cooked	4	Kidney beans, ½ cup, cooked	3
Chicken leg, 4 ounces, cooked	2	Tofu cubes, ½ cup	3
Pork, 4 ounces, cooked	1		
Chicken breast, 4 ounces, cooked	1	**Grains**	
Salmon, 4 ounces, cooked	1	Cereal, 100% iron fortified, 1 cup	18
Egg, 1 large	1	Spaghetti, 1 cup, cooked	2
		Bread, enriched, 1 slice	1
Fruits		**Other**	
Prunes, 5	1	Molasses, blackstrap, 1 tablespoon	3
Raisins, ⅓ cup	1		
Dried apricots, ⅓ cup	1	Wheat germ, ¼ cup	2

1 cup = 240 milliliters; 1 tablespoon = 15 milliliters; 1 ounce = 28 grams; 4 ounces = 112 grams

Nutrition information from food labels, USDA National Nutrient Database (online), and J. Pennington, 2004, Bowes & Church's Food Values of Portions Commonly Used, 18th ed. (Philadelphia: Lippincott, Williams & Wilkins)

The recommended intake for zinc is 8 milligrams for women and 11 milligrams for men per day. Animal foods, including seafood, are the best sources of zinc.

Animal Sources (best absorbed)	Zinc (mg)	Plant Sources	Zinc (mg)
		Wheat germ, ¼ cup	3
Beef tenderloin, 4 ounces cooked	7	Lentils, 1 cup cooked	2
Chicken leg, 4 ounces cooked	4	Almonds, 1 ounce	1
Pork loin, 4 ounces cooked	3	Garbanzo beans, ½ cup	1
Chicken breast, 4 ounces cooked	1	Spinach, 1 cup cooked	1
Cheese, 1 ounce	1	Peanut butter, 1 tablespoon	0.5
Milk, 1 cup	1	Bread, 1 slice, whole wheat	0.5
Oysters, 6 medium	(!) 75	1 cup = 240 milliliters;	
Tuna, 1 can (6.5 ounces)	2	1 tablespoon = 15 milliliters;	
Clams, 9 small	1	1 ounce = 28 grams; 4 ounces = 112 grams	

Meat and Zinc   Ordinarily, foods rich in iron are also rich in zinc, and red meat is no exception. If you don't eat meat or if you eat an iron-poor diet, chances are your diet is lacking in zinc. Zinc is important for healing minor, day-to-day tissue damage as well as major injuries and ailments. Like iron, the zinc in red meat and other animal protein is better absorbed than the zinc in plant foods or supplements.

Hormones and Antibiotics in Meats—Fears abound regarding hormones given to cattle to enhance their growth and health. You can always buy "all-natural" or organic meat to be on the safe side. Yet, the U.S. Department of Agriculture claims the amount of hormones used is far less than one might get in a birth control pill, or even in a cup of coleslaw, for that matter. The use of antibiotics to keep the animals healthy may be a valid concern; this practice may be implicated in the rising incidence of antibiotic resistance in the U.S.

● SUMMARY—
● Most cyclists have hearty appetites and end up eating more than enough protein.
● Contrary to popular notion, eating a lot of protein does not

enhance muscle growth, strength, or size. The best way to build muscle and strength is through resistance training and a wholesome, carbohydrate-rich diet.

- A protein-poor diet can lead to fatigue, anemia, lack of athletic improvement, muscle wasting, and an overall run-down feeling. Iron and zinc deficiencies can occur with a protein-poor diet, since these minerals are found primarily in protein-rich foods.

- To meet their protein needs, a vegetarians should eat a variety of protein-rich plant foods.

- To eat meat or not is a personal choice. You need not feel guilty if you eat red meat, nor should you feel righteous if you choose tofu. Cyclists can enjoy both types of diets in good health, if they choose wisely. The trick is to consume adequate protein, iron, zinc, and other nutrients by eating a variety of wholesome foods that are low in saturated fat.

CHAPTER 6

Fats and Your Sports Diet

MANY CYCLISTS RESTRICT THEIR FAT INTAKE BECAUSE OF THEIR desire to be healthy. This is a wise health practice that is often taken to the extreme. Some cyclists think all they need to know about fat is that it is bad and they are supposed to avoid it. Rumors abound:

- Fat instantly clogs the arteries.
- Fat causes cancer.
- Fat is the worst food you could put in your body.
- If you eat fat, you'll get fat.

While there is an element of truth in these statements, they are mostly inaccurate.

Other cyclists pay no attention to fat in their diets, especially when they are riding. They may think they burn off all the fat they eat as they pedal down the road. Or they may believe they have earned a post-ride meal of cheeseburgers, pepperoni pizza, or ice cream. Whereas a little bit of fat is an appropriate part of a sports diet, too much fat is not:

- A high-fat diet can lack carbohydrates, leaving your muscles unfueled.
- A diet saturated with animal and hydrogenated fats contributes to heart disease and cancer and may shorten your life span.
- Fat has over twice the calories of protein or carbohydrate, so excess fat calories can add up easily and lead to weight gain.

Cyclists who eat too much fat would do better to substitute some of their fat calories for more carbohydrate calories.

As you plan your healthful sports diet, remember that fat is

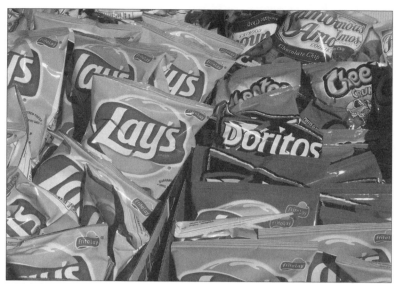

A high-fat diet can lack carbohydrates, leaving your muscles unfueled. Healthy cyclists should target a 25-percent-fat diet by rationing their intake of obviously fatty foods. Baked chips, please.

an essential nutrient needed for overall good health and optimal performance. The fat you eat helps to carry fat-soluble nutrients, such as vitamins A, D, E, and K, and carotenoids, from your intestines into your bloodstream. Certain fats contain essential fatty acids, which your body requires but cannot make. Essential fatty acids are necessary for good health: growth, cell repair, nerve function, and immune function. Eating certain types of fats—like the monounsaturated and polyunsaturated fats found in nuts, flaxseed, fish, and olives— may reduce your risk of certain diseases, particularly heart disease. And long-distance cyclists who include some fat in their daily training diet are more likely to enjoy greater stamina and endurance than those who try to exclude fat.

● **HOW MUCH FAT SHOULD YOU EAT?**—If you are lean, fit, and healthy and you have low or normal blood cholesterol (or high levels of the good HDL cholesterol), a family history of longevity, and no family history of heart disease, you can appropriately include and enjoy a reasonable amount of fat in your diet. The people who most likely need to restrict their fat intake to very limited amounts are over-fat, under-fit folks at high risk for heart disease, not most healthy cyclists.

Most healthy cyclists can target a sports diet with about 25 percent of the calories from fat. This amount of fat:

- is consistent with the 20 percent to 35 percent fat diet that is considered to be health-protective;
- gives you enough carbohydrates (55 percent to 65 percent of total calories) for restoring muscle glycogen and enough protein (10 percent to 15 percent of total calories) for muscle maintenance and repair;
- provides fat for storage within the muscles and gets used during extended bike rides;
- provides essential fatty acids and fat-soluble vitamins;
- allows for easier participation in life (i.e., eating at a party, enjoying a cookie guilt-free); and
- gives you enough fat for taste and good nutrition without providing excess calories that contribute to weight gain.

How does a 25-percent-fat diet translate into food? A cyclist who eats 2,800 calories a day could eat 700 calories from fat or about 75 grams of fat a day:

Multiply a daily calorie budget of 2,800 calories by 25 percent:
2,800 total calories x 0.25 = 700 calories a day of fat.

Because there are nine calories per gram of fat,
divide 700 calories by nine:
700 calories / 9 calories per gram =
75 grams of fat in your daily fat budget.

For your daily calorie budget, see chapter 13. See the guidelines for fat on page 64 to estimate how many fat grams you should target per day.

● **HEALTHFUL FATS**—You can easily achieve a diet that is 25 percent fat by rationing your intake of obviously fatty foods (fried foods, butter, greasy meats, salad dressings, etc.), but you should also pay attention to the kinds of fat you eat. The majority of the fat in your diet should consist of health-protective monounsaturated and polyunsaturated fats, such as those found in olive oil, canola oil, nuts, peanut butter, and oily fish.

To reduce your risk of heart disease, you should eat a lesser amount of saturated and trans (hydrogenated and partially hydrogenated) fats, such as those found in animal fat (meat,

The following guidelines can help you appropriately include fat in your food plan.

Calories per day	Fat grams per day (for a 25-percent-fat diet)
1,800	50
2,000	55
2,200	60
2,400	65
2,600	70
2,800	75
3,000	85

Fat and Calories in Common Foods

Food	Amount	Fat (g)	Cal.	Food	Amount	Fat (g)	Cal.
Milk products				Ice cream, gourmet	½ cup	15	250
Milk, whole (3½% fat)	1 cup	8	150	Ice cream, light	½ cup	3	110
Milk, low-fat (1%, ½% fat)	1 cup	2	100	Frozen yogurt, low-fat	½ cup	2	120
Milk, fat-free	1 cup	—	80	**Animal proteins (cooked)**			
Cheddar cheese	1 oz.	9	110	Beef, hamburger	4 oz.	24	330
Cheddar cheese, reduced-fat	1 oz.	5	90	Top sirloin	4 oz.	10	240
				Chicken, breast,	4 oz.	5	200
Cottage cheese (4% fat)	½ cup	5	120	Chicken thigh, no skin	4 oz.	11	235
Cottage cheese Low-fat (2% fat)	½ cup	2	90	Haddock	4 oz.	1	125
				Swordfish	4 oz.	6	175
Cream cheese	2 T	10	100	**Fruits and vegetables**			
Cream cheese, light	2 T	5	60	most varieties		negligible fat	

cheese, butter), fried foods (chips, donuts, fried chicken), stick margarine, and baked goods (muffins, pie crust, cookies). If you enjoy eating some of these foods (and most hungry cyclists do), the healthy thing to do is to eat them in moderation and balance them into your weekly calorie and fat budget. For example, when you have the occasional hankering for a burger and fries, indulge. But balance out your day, and the next day if necessary, with plenty of fruits, vegetables, and low-fat foods.

Making simple substitutions in food choices throughout the day can make a healthier diet. Even when you are touring, you can try to swap foods rich in "bad fat" with those that contain more "good fats" (see chart on page 66).

Fat and Calories in Common Foods

Food	Amount	Fat (g)	Cal.
Vegetable proteins			
Beans, kidney cooked	½ cup	—	110
Tofu	4 oz.	5	90
Peanut butter	1 T	8	95
Mixed nuts	1 oz. or 3 T	15	170
Fats			
Butter, Margarine	1 T	12	105
Oil, olive	1 T	13	120
Mayonnaise	1 T	11	100
Grains			
Bread, large slice whole wheat	1	1	90
Saltines	5	2	60
Ritz	4	4	70
Rice cakes	1	—	35
Shredded wheat	²/₃ cup	—	90
Granola	¼ cup	6	130
Oatmeal, cooked	²/₃ cup	2	100

Food	Amount	Fat (g)	Cal.
Spaghetti	1 cup cooked	1	210
Rice	1 cup cooked	—	200
Fast foods			
Big Mac	1	30	570
Egg McMuffin	1	12	290
French fries	small	10	210
Fried chicken	1 breast	24	400
Pizza, cheese	1 slice	10-13	250
Snacks, treats			
Cookie, Chips Ahoy	1	2	50
Fig Newton	1	1	60
Brownie, from mix	1 small	5	140
Graham crackers	2 squares	1	60
Potato chips	18 (1 oz.)	9	150
Pretzels	1 oz.	1	110
Milky Way	1.75-oz. bar	8	220
M&Ms with peanuts	1.75-oz. bag	13	250

1 cup = 240 milliliters; 1 tablespoon = 15 milliliters; 1 ounce = 28 grams; 4 ounces = 112 grams

Nutrition information from food labels, USDA National Nutrient Database (online), and J. Pennington, 2004, Bowes & Church's Food Values of Portions Commonly Used, 18th ed. (Philadelphia: Lippincott, Williams & Wilkins)

• **FEAR OF FAT**—Without a doubt, fat imparts a tempting taste, texture, and aroma and helps make food delicious. That's why fatty foods can be hard to resist and are often enjoyed to excess. Although excess calories from fat can easily turn into body fat, the eat-fat-get-fat theory is false. What does add to body fat is eating excess *calories*—not just from fat but also from protein, carbohydrate, and alcohol. Many cyclists eat appropriate amounts of fat and stay thin. They simply don't overeat calories.

If you are weight-conscious and obsess about every gram of fat to the extent you have a fat phobia, your fear of fat may be exaggerated! A little fat can actually aid in weight reduction.

Meal	Instead of these (rich in saturated or trans fat):	Choose these (rich in mono- and/or poly-unsaturated fat):
Breakfast	Croissant	Bagel with peanut butter
	Cheese omelet	Vegetable omelet
	Donut	Whole-wheat toast with almond butter
	Muffin	Handful of cereal with raisins and nuts added
Lunch	Roast beef sandwich	Peanut butter sandwich
	Turkey and cheese sub	Tuna sub made with mayonnaise, preferably reduced-fat
	Roll-up with cheese and veggies	Roll-up with hummus, veggies
	Cheese on a salad or sandwich	Avocado or olives on a salad or sandwich
	Deli meat	Canned sardines or tuna
Snack	Cheese	Almonds or olives
	Packaged cookies or chocolate	Dried fruit and nut mix
Dinner	Blue cheese salad dressing	Vinaigrette or Italian dressing
	Butter on a roll	Olive oil on a roll
	Steak	Grilled fish
	Fettuccini with alfredo sauce	Fettuccine with garlic, olive oil
	Spaghetti with meat balls	Spaghetti with clam sauce
	Hamburger	Veggie or salmon burger
	Vanilla ice cream	Low-fat frozen yogurt sprinkled with nuts

Dietary fat contributes to the nice feeling of being satisfied after a meal, and may help you eat less during and after a meal. If you have the desire to continue eating even after you've eaten an unsatisfying fat-free meal, try adding a little more fat to your diet. Refer to the weight reduction information in chapter 14 for additional help with resolving your eat-fat-get-fat fears.

● SUMMARY—

- Eating too much fat can lead to unfueled muscles and excess calories and weight gain.
- The key to eating the right amount of fat is moderation: a wholesome diet that includes about 25 percent of the calories

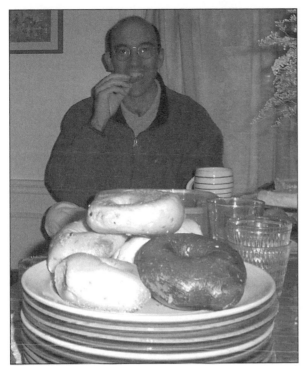

Spreading peanut butter on a bagel adds more protein and healthful fat than you'd get from cream cheese or butter.

as fat. This translates into a little fat each meal or one fatty meal per day.

- For optimum health, choose healthful mono- and poly-unsaturated fats (olive oil, vegetable oils, nuts, fish) more often than saturated and trans fat (fried foods, bakery treats, and greasy burgers).
- All fats—even your favorite burger and the occasional order of French fries—eaten in moderation can be balanced into an overall healthful and carbohydrate-based sports diet.

CHAPTER 7

Water, Sports Drinks, and Other Fluids

WATER IS AN ESSENTIAL NUTRIENT AS EQUALLY IMPORTANT AS carbohydrates, proteins, and fats. Cyclists need adequate water for body fluids:

- Sweat to dissipate heat
- Urine to help carry away the waste products
- Blood to help carry oxygen and fuel to working muscles
- Body fluids to lubricate joints, muscles, and tissues
- Gastric juices to digest food

Sweating accounts for the majority of fluids lost during cycling. During hard exercise, your muscles can generate 15 to 20 times more heat than they do when you are at rest. Sweating is your body's way of dissipating this heat and keeping you from overheating. Evaporating sweat cools your skin. This in turn cools the blood and reduces your body temperature. Some cyclists sweat profusely, soaking their helmets and riding jerseys (and sometimes showering the riders drafting behind them!) even on shorter rides. Others seem to barely sweat at all. In dryer climates and colder weather, you may not feel like you sweat as much, but you still lose fluids while exercising. All cyclists in all climates in all seasons need to be attentive to replacing sweat losses.

66*I'm very diligent about keeping myself hydrated...there's nothing worse than crossing the finish line with the driest tongue stuck to your mouth!* **99**

Kate Riedell, Fairfield, CT

- **HOW MUCH SHOULD YOU DRINK?**—The American College of Sports Medicine recom-

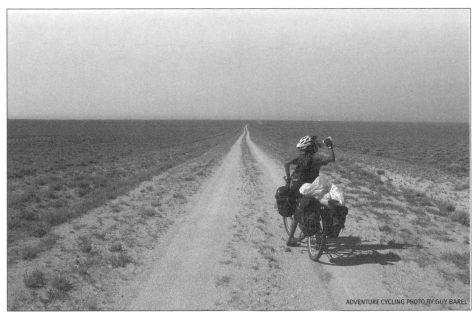

When you are faced with a long road ahead of you and no known water source, tank up beforehand, carry extra water and take frequent water stops.

mends drinking four to eight ounces (120 to 240 milliliters) of fluid every 15 to 20 minutes during hard exercise, but it varies by individual. For optimal hydration, you should balance your fluid losses with your fluid intake as you go along. To determine how much fluid you lose while biking, in other words, your "sweat rate," weigh yourself naked before and after one hour of training without eating or drinking. Replace the amount of weight you have lost with equal amounts of water. For every pound you have lost, you need to drink a pound (or 16 ounces)

> **❝On long, hot rides, I have done a dual Camelbak approach where I put water in one bladder and a sports drink in the other. ❞**
>
> Doug Davis, Dallas, TX

of water. Or for every kilogram lost, drink one liter of water. So if your sweat rate is two pounds (or approximately one kilogram) per hour, you should plan to drink 32 ounces (one liter) every hour while riding—ideally, eight ounces (240 milliliters) every fifteen minutes.

Cyclists who fail to replace fluid losses can suffer from chronic dehydration. Dehydration slows you down, contributes to needless fatigue and lethargy, and in extreme cases, contributes to medical problems. You can tell if you are well-

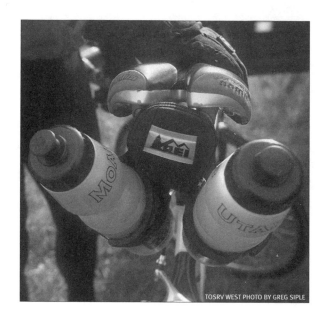

TOSRV WEST PHOTO BY GREG SIPLE

Depending on your sweat rate, you should plan to drink about one large bike bottle (24 ounces) per hour during a ride.

hydrated by monitoring your urine:

- You should urinate frequently (every two to four hours) throughout the day.
- The urine should be clear, pale yellow, and of significant quantity.
- Your morning urine should not be dark and concentrated.
- Your urine may be dark yellow if you take multivitamin supplements. In this case, volume of urine is a better indicator of hydration than is color.

Many cyclists make the mistake of waiting until they are thirsty to drink, but when you reach this point, you are already dehydrated. By the time your brain signals thirst, you may have lost 1 percent or more of your body weight, the equivalent of 24 ounces (675 milliliters) of sweat for a cyclist who weighs 150 pounds (70 kilograms). A 1 percent sweat loss can cause your heart to beat an extra three to five times per minute (Casa et al. 2000). An increased heart rate increases your breathing rate, so you feel like you are working harder. A 3 percent sweat loss can significantly hurt your performance. You should strive to lose no more than 2 percent of your body weight per exercise session.

Because the sensation of thirst is an unreliable indicator to drink, you should program your drinking according to your

A pound of sweat contains about 80 to 100 milligrams of potassium and 400 to 700 milligrams of sodium. In two hours of moderately sweaty riding, you might burn 1,200 calories and lose 32 ounces (900 milliliters) of water, 400 milligrams of potassium, and 3,000 milligrams of sodium in your sweat. To help you recover these losses, you can choose from these popular sports foods and beverages.

Fluid Per 8 oz./240 ml	Calories	Carb. (g)	Sodium (mg)	Potassium (mg)
Water	0	0	0	0
Gatorade	50	14	110	30
Powerade	70	19	55	30
Cytomax	70	15	75	80
Accelerade	90	17	125	40
Cola	100	25	5	—
Beer	100	7	12	60
Light beer	65	3	6	40
Orange juice	110	25	2	475
Cranberry apple juice drink	165	40	5	65
Low-fat milk	100	12	125	380
Chocolate low-fat milk	160	25	150	425
V8 juice	50	10	737	512
Vegetable soup, canned	120	20	1,010	395
Fruit yogurt (low-fat)	225	40	120	400

Nutrition information from food labels, product websites, and J. Pennington, 2004, Bowes & Church's Food Values of Portions Commonly Used, 18th ed. (Philadelphia: Lippincott, Williams & Wilkins)

sweat rate. Plan to drink on a schedule so that you do not fall short of your fluid goals. For example, drink four gulps (roughly 4 ounces or 120 milliliters) every 15 minutes or every few miles. Practice drinking during training rides to become familiar with the skills involved in drinking while riding as well as your body's capacity for fluids. Also try different sports drinks, juices, and other beverages during training to see which of them you prefer and which of them you best tolerate. When you get off the bike, drink enough to quench your thirst, plus more just to be safe.

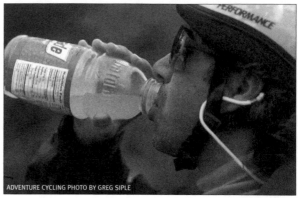

ADVENTURE CYCLING PHOTO BY GREG SIPLE

Sports drinks come in many flavors and brands. Experiment during training rides to find the one that suit you best.

● **SPORTS DRINKS**—During bike tours, events, and training sessions that last longer than 60 to 90 minutes, you will perform better if you consume more than just plain water. If you are not going to be eating solid food, sports drinks can provide:

- small amounts of carbohydrates to fuel your mind and muscles,
- sodium and potassium to enhance water absorption and retention, and
- water to replace fluid losses.

With the multitude of sports drinks available today, it is easy to feel confused about what's best to drink. The beverage perfect for all athletes in all events has yet to be designed. There are enormous individual differences among people's stomach function and therefore their tolerance to food and fluid during exercise. This helps to explain why some people seek out or avoid a particular brand of sports drink and some can drink just about anything. Basically there are no significant advantages to one sports drink over another. The best sport beverage is the one that you prefer to drink, and the one you'll drink plenty of! And remember, any fluid, be it water or sports drink, is better than no fluid during extended exercise.

The average male's body contains about 75,000 milligrams of sodium, the amount found in 11 tablespoons of salt. A pound (16 ounces) of sweat contains 400 to 700 milligrams of sodium. In an hour of riding you may lose 400 to 1,500 milligrams, depending on:

How much you sweat. The more you sweat, the more sodium you can lose.

How much salt you eat. The more salt you eat, the more salt you lose in sweat.

How much you exercise In the heat and how fit you are. If you are fit and heat acclimatized, you will conserve sodium to defend against sodium depletion.

You can easily replace the sodium losses by eating some of these popular recovery foods:

Food	Sodium (mg)	Food	Sodium (mg)
Pizza, ¹/₂ medium	1,400	Vegetable soup,	
Spaghetti sauce, 1 cup	750	1 cup	1,200
Muffin, 1 medium	500	Salt, 1 packet	500
Saltines, 10	400	Salt, ¹/₄ teaspoon	575

Although sports drinks are thought to be a sodium-rich recovery beverage, they are actually sodium-poor, containing only 50 to 110 milligrams per 8 ounces. For more foods and fluids, see *Comparing Fluid Replacers* on page 71.

Nutrition information from food labels and J. Pennington, 2004, Bowes & Church's Food Values of Portions Commonly Used, 18th ed. (Philadelphia: Lippincott, Williams & Wilkins).

● **ELECTROLYTE REPLACEMENT**—When you sweat, you lose electrolytes, such as sodium and potassium, two of the minerals that help maintain proper water balance in your tissues. Contrary to what many athletes think, commercial sports drinks include these electrolytes not to replace those lost in sweat, but primarily to increase the absorption rate of the water into your body.

Most cyclists who ride or race for a couple of hours do not have to worry about replacing electrolytes during exercise because the losses are generally too small to cause a deficit that will hurt performance and/or health. But, for exercise that lasts four hours or more, occurs in very hot weather, or goes on for several days (randonnée, tour, stage race) electrolyte losses can become problematic, particularly if you are

❝I have found when I drink sports drinks I finish stronger than my friends who drink only water. ❞

Lenny Sullivan, Methuen, MA

drinking mostly water during that time. Drinking too much plain water during extended, sweaty exercise can create an electrolyte imbalance in your body. In particular, a low level of sodium in the body, or hyponatremia, causes fatigue, nausea, headache, cramps, and diarrhea. If left unchecked, hyponatremia can lead to confusion, poor coordination, seizures, and even death.

If you plan to ride hard for more than four hours, also plan to consume sodium and potassium during the ride. Give up plain water and have fluids and foods that contain some sodium and potassium, such as sports drinks, energy bars, tomato juice, pretzels, salted nuts, and fig bars. If you're on a tour or randonnée that lasts for several days, be extra careful to include salty foods in your daily meal plan, for example, salt in your morning oatmeal, mustard on your lunchtime sandwich, and soup or tomato sauce with dinner. See *Comparing Fluid Replacers* on page 71 and *How Much Sodium Do You Lose in Sweat?* on page 73 for information on popular fluids and foods.

• **HOW TO KEEP YOUR COOL**—The following true-false quiz will test your knowledge about fluid replacement and will help you survive the heat in good health and with high energy.

Drinking cold water during exercise will cool you off.—True, but only by a small margin. Although drinking cold water will cool you off slightly more than warmer water, the difference is small because the water quickly warms to body temperature. The more important concern is quantity. Any fluid of any temperature is better than no fluid.

Despite popular belief, salt for athletes is not a four-letter word. The public health recommendations to reduce salt intake are directed to people who are overweight, under-fit, and have high blood pressure, not lean, fit cyclists with normal or low blood pressure.

How much salt do cyclists actually need?

Salt (or more correctly sodium, the part of salt that is the health culprit) requirements depend upon how much you sweat. A "safe and adequate" sodium intake for the average person is 2,400 milligrams per day. The typical American intake is 3,000 to 6,000 milligrams of sodium per day, which tends to cover the sodium needs of most cyclists.

- The rule of thumb is to add extra salt to your diet if you have lost more than 4 to 6 pounds of sweat (3-4 percent of your body weight pre- to post-ride).
- Too little salt can result in fatigue and muscle cramps.
- Cyclists who sweat profusely day after day and eat primarily low-salt foods may benefit from adding a little sodium to replace that lost in sweat, particularly if muscle cramps are a problem.
- If you'll be riding for longer than four hours, drink and/or eat foods that contain added salt, such as sodium-containing sports drinks, pretzels, cheese (in a sandwich), vegetable juices, soups, and energy bars.

If I crave salt, should I eat it?

Yes. Salt cravings signal that your body wants salt. If you hanker for some pretzels or salty foods, eat them!

Drinking water 30 minutes before exercise eliminates the need to drink fluids during a long training session.—False. Research suggests that drinking a quart of water before exercise is less effective than drinking an equal volume during exercise. Researchers aren't sure why, but they recommend the optimal approach: Tank up beforehand plus drink enough to match your sweat losses during exercise.

Soda is a poor choice during exercise because the carbon dioxide in the bubbles will slow you down.—False. Historically, athletes were always warned to "de-fizz" carbonated beverages taken during exercise, fearing that the carbonation would interfere with oxygen transport, upset the stomach,

Homemade Sports Drink

After water, the main ingredients in commercial fluid replacers (sports drinks) are sugar, sodium, and potassium. Eight ounces (240 milliliters) of sports drink contains about:

- 3 teaspoons, of sugar (50 calories);
- 50 to 110 milligrams of sodium, equal to about $^1/_{16}$ teaspoon or 1 pinch of salt; and
- 30 to 50 milligrams of potassium.

The following recipe provides the same nutrition profile, but at a much lower cost than commercial brands.

¼ cup sugar

¼ teaspoon salt

¼ cup hot water

¼ cup orange juice (not concentrate)

3½ cups cold water

1. In a 1-quart (or 1-liter) bottle with a cover, dissolve the sugar and salt in the hot water.

2. Add the juices and cold water. Cover. Shake well.

3. Quench that thirst!

YIELD:	1 quart or
	4 (8-oz. or 240-ml) servings

Nutrition Information

TOTAL CALORIES:	200
CALORIES PER SERVING:	50

Nutrient	Grams per serving
CARBOHYDRATE	12
PROTEIN	—
FAT	—
SODIUM	110 mg
POTASSIUM	30 mg

1 cup = 240 milliliters; 1 tablespoon = 15 milliliters; 1 ounce = 28 grams; 4 ounces = 112 grams

and hurt performance. New studies comparing carbonated and non-carbonated soft drinks show bubbles will not hurt your performance nor result in stomach discomfort.

Don't bother to drink during a ride that is shorter than an hour because the fluid has too little time to get into your system.— False. According to Larry Armstrong, exercise physiologist at the University of Connecticut, water can travel from stomach to skin in just nine to 18 minutes after drinking. This water is essential for dissipating the heat you produce during exercise. Your best bet is to try to match sweat losses with an equal volume of fluid intake during exercise, even if it's under an hour.

Beer is an appropriate recovery fluid.—False. Although beer is a popular recovery drink, it lacks what your depleted body needs after exercise. If you are not accustomed to drinking beer, it will have a dehydrating effect, and so it's a poor source of fluid. Beer and most other alcoholic beverages are also poor sources of carbohydrates. A twelve-ounce (360-milliliter) bottle of beer has only 14 grams of carbohydrates; the same amount of juice or cola has 40 grams. And, alcohol acts as a depressant. If you drink alcohol on an empty stomach, as commonly happens post-race, you quickly can negate the pleasurable "natural high" that you would otherwise enjoy. Wise beer-drinkers first have one or two glasses of water and eat some carbohydrate-rich foods (pretzels, pizza, crackers), and then they enjoy a beer or two in moderation.

66 *When pounding down a lot of water on those hot, humid days, I have to be careful to take some salty stuff like V-8 juice. Otherwise, I'll begin to feel the effects of sodium depletion.* **99**

Ed Kross, Framingham, MA

• SUMMARY—

- For optimal hydration, you should tank up before riding and drink enough to match your sweat losses during the ride, generally four to eight ounces (120 to 240 milliliters) of fluid every 15 to 20 minutes.
- If you'll be riding longer than 60 to 90 minutes, you will perform better if you consume a source of carbohydrates and fluid.
- Commercial sports drinks include sodium, not to replace that lost in sweat, but primarily to increase the absorption rate of the water into your body.
- Most cyclists who ride or race for a couple of hours do not have to worry about replacing electrolytes during exercise. If you plan to ride for more than four hours or all day long, plan to consume sodium and potassium during the ride.

CHAPTER 8

Fueling Before You Ride

EATING BEFORE RIDING PROMISES ADVANTAGES THAT CONTRIBUTE TO better performance, more energy and stamina, and faster recovery. But food and drink can sometimes be a problem for people who fear upset stomachs, abdominal cramps, and bathroom stops that interfere with riding. This chapter provides useful information about pre-exercise food and drink to help you devise a pre-ride nutrition strategy that will maximize your performance and enjoyment during every ride.

> **❝I have learned many things about my body. Initially, I couldn't eat before exercise or else I would get nauseated. Realizing I needed energy before heading out, I finally discovered that a glass of milk kick-starts me without ill effects. ❞**
>
> Kim Holland, Maitland, FL

● **BENEFITS OF PRE-RIDE FOOD**—Research demonstrates that eating more carbohydrates (or carbo-loading) the days before an event maximizes muscle glycogen stores and improves performance in events lasting 90 minutes or more. Consuming carbohydrates three to four hours before exercise tops off liver and muscle glycogen stores and enhances endurance performance (Hargreaves et al. 2004).

For touring cyclists, this advantage can mean the difference between fully enjoying or barely enduring a day of riding. For competitive cyclists, it can mean the difference between a podium finish and getting dropped by the pack. Here are some helpful facts to give you some insight about the benefits of eating before riding.

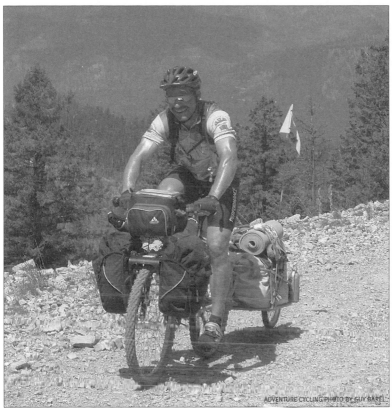

Without question, breakfast is essential to boost your blood sugar and fuel your body's engine for a long day of riding.

1. Pre-ride carbohydrates fuel the muscles.—Your body has approximately 1,800 calories worth of carbohydrates (or glucose) stored as glycogen in the muscles (1,400 calories) and liver (350 calories). These limited stores influence how long and how hard you can enjoy riding. When your glycogen stores get too low, your body will feel utterly exhausted, you'll yearn to stop, and your performance (and morale) will rapidly decline. This is commonly referred to as "hitting the wall."

In contrast to your very limited glycogen stores, you have nearly 100,000 calories worth of fat in your body. Unfortunately for endurance cyclists, the body cannot use just fat to fuel itself; it requires some carbohydrate to burn fat. In the absence of carbohydrates your body will begin to break down muscle protein for energy.

The carbs you eat even an hour before riding are digested and converted to glucose to:
1) top off your glycogen stores,
2) be used for energy by muscles, thereby sparing your glycogen stores, and thus
3) delay the onset of fatigue.

2. Pre-ride food helps prevent low blood sugar (hypoglycemia).— When your muscles are depleted of glycogen, you hit the wall; when your blood sugar (glucose) levels drop, you bonk. The two often happen simultaneously.

The brain requires a steady supply of glucose (stored in the liver) for fuel. When the liver glycogen runs low, your blood sugar will drop, your brain will be deprived of adequate glucose, and you will begin to feel the effects of hypoglycemia: lightheadedness, irritability, blurred vision, sleepiness, and inability to think clearly. A poorly fueled brain also impairs muscle function and mental drive. One racer (now a pro racer and coach) once bonked so badly he got off his bike, wandered over to some shady grass, and took a nap for one of the laps in the middle of a road race (obviously not only sleepy but also judgment-impaired)! To prevent the dreaded bonk, you need both pre-ride carbohydrates and a steady supply during rides.

If you ride first thing in the morning with nothing to eat, be aware that you have essentially fasted since dinnertime the evening before and you likely could improve your stamina and mental drive by consuming some carbohydrates before heading out. Some early morning riders consume nothing yet report that they have plenty of energy. Most likely, they ate a substantial dinner and/or serious late-night snack the night before, which bolsters liver glycogen stores and reduces the need for a morning energizer. This is not bad or wrong as long as this pattern works well for them.

Historically, athletes were told to choose starchy complex carbohydrates such as pasta for the pre-ride meal in preference to sugary simple carbohydrates such as soft drinks. The theory was that starches would contribute to a stable blood sugar level and sugary carbohydrates would contribute to a sugar high following by a sugar low and debilitating hypoglycemia. Today, we know that cyclists should not choose their pre-ride carbo-

The following list ranks foods according to their ability to elevate blood sugar given a 200-calorie (50-gram) dose of carbohydrates. Many factors influence the glycemic effect of a food, such as what you eat with the food, meal size, and food preparation. Foods ranked over 70 are considered to have a high glycemic index; foods ranked lower than 40 have a low glycemic index.

High					
Glucose	100	Snickers	68	Grapes	46
Dates, dried	100	Chocolate ice cream	68	Spaghetti, plain	44
Cornflakes	92	Cream of Wheat, reg.	66	Lentil soup	44
Honey	87	Oatmeal	66	Chocolate milk	43
Potato, baked	85	Powerade	65	Orange	42
Shredded wheat	83	Couscous	65	*Low*	
Pretzels	81	Raisins	64	Apple juice, unsweetened	40
Gatorade	78	Coca-Cola	63	PR-Bar, Ironman chocolate	39
Cheerios	74	Cytomax	62	All-Bran cereal	38
Graham crackers	74	Raisin Bran	61	Apple	38
Bread, whole-wheat	73	Sweet potato	61	Ice cream	36
Bagel, white	72	Corn	60	Chocolate milk	34
Watermelon	72	Cheese pizza	60	Fruit yogurt	33
Grape-Nuts	71	Peanut butter sandwich	60	M&Ms, Peanut	33
Bread, white	70	PowerBar, chocolate	58	Milk, fat-free	32
Skittles	70	Rice, white boiled	58	Lentils, boiled	30
Moderate		Rice, brown	55	Peach	28
Soft drink, Fanta	68	Banana	52	Milk, whole	27
Sugar, white (sucrose)	68	Kidney beans	52	Grapefruit	25
Cranberry juice	68	Peas, green	48	Peanuts	15
		Orange Juice	46		

Data from food companies; Foster-Powell et al. 2002; and Gretebeck et al. 2002; and http://diabetes.about.com/library/mendosagi/ngilists.htm.

hydrates based on whether they are complex or simple, but experiment with carbohydrates based on their glycemic index.

The glycemic index ranks foods according to their ability to contribute glucose into the bloodstream (see *Glycemic Index of Common Sports Foods* above).

- Low glycemic foods are desirable before a long ride because they are digested and absorbed into the bloodstream slowly, providing sustained energy, and more stable blood sugar.

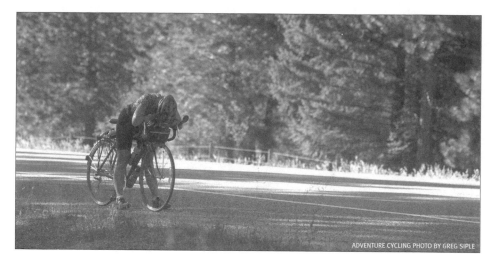

To prevent bonking, consume carbohydrate-based meals and snacks on a daily basis, and consume carbohydrates before and during your ride.

> **My worst nutrition error was assuming that lower is better when it comes to the glycemic index. While it follows that oatmeal is preferable to Froot Loops, it does not follow that lentils make a better choice than oatmeal. I once ruined 30 miles of a 100-miler with the worst stomach cramps after consuming a bowl of curried lentils for breakfast!**
>
> Stuart Boyd, Wilmington, MA

- High glycemic index foods quickly elevate blood sugar. They can initiate hypoglycemic reactions in people sensitive to swings in blood sugar. Foods with a high glycemic index are preferable for recovery foods, when your depleted muscles readily absorb all available glucose.

A recent study showed that cyclists who ate 300 calories of carbohydrates from oatmeal (a moderate glycemic index food) before riding were able to ride hard for longer than those who ate the same calories from puffed rice (high glycemic index) (Kirwan et al. 2001). But other such studies failed to demonstrate similar results (Wee et al. 1999). This may be explained by individual glycemic responses to foods. Your best bet is to experiment during training. For instance, if you have been eating a pre-exercise microwaved potato, try a fruit yogurt to see if it contributes to better performance. Keep in mind: rather than fret about what to eat before a long ride, know that *fueling during the ride* is the better way to enhance stamina and endurance.

To be sufficiently fueled for long training rides, hard workouts, races, or all-day riding events, you should do minimal exercise the day before and plan your meals according to this schedule. Always drink additional fluids with and between meals to ensure complete hydration. If you tend to be overly nervous or have a sensitive stomach prior to a stressful event, you may want to limit your food intake on that day and make a special effort to eat extra food the day before. If you are on a bike tour, you need to wisely eat and drink throughout the day to invest in sustained energy for the length of the tour.

Morning event
Day before: Eat a hearty, high-carbohydrate lunch, dinner, and bedtime snack.
Event day: Eat a comfortable, carbohydrate-rich snack/breakfast to abate hunger feelings, and get your blood glucose on the upswing.

Afternoon event
Day before: Eat a hearty, high-carbohydrate dinner.
Event day: Eat a hearty high-carbohydrate breakfast and a comfortable lunch, as tolerated.

Evening event
Event day: Eat a hearty, high-carbohydrate breakfast and lunch.
Eat a comfortable, carbohydrate-rich snack 1 to 3 hours prior to the event, as tolerated.

3. Pre-ride food helps settle the stomach, absorbs some of the gastric juices, and abates hunger.- For many people, the stress associated with competition or other cycling events stimulates gastric secretions and contributes to an acid stomach. Eating a small amount of food can help alleviate that problem. Eating 100 to 300 calories of a low-fat, carbohydrate-rich snack within the hour before riding will provide fuel and should sit comfortably in your stomach. Try eating a small bowl of oatmeal, half a bagel, a few crackers. You'll learn by trial and error what foods work, what ones don't.

4. Pre-ride beverages can provide fluids to fully hydrate your body as well as additional carbohydrates.—By tanking up on sports drinks or diluted juice before you ride, you can help prevent dehydration and also boost your carbohydrate and energy intake. You should drink plenty of fluids every day whether you ride or not, in both hot and cold weather. You can confirm you have had enough to drink by frequent urination and clear-colored urine. If your urine is dark and concentrated, you need more fluids. Refer to the previous chapter for more information on hydration.

5. Pre-ride food can pacify your mind with the knowledge that your body is well-fueled.— Before a long ride or race, you don't want to waste any energy wondering if you have eaten enough. Appropriate eating can resolve that concern! Pre-exercise food has great psychological value. If you firmly believe that a specific food will enhance your performance, then it probably will. Your mind has a powerful effect on your body's ability to perform at its best. If you have a magic food that assures athletic excellence, you should take special care to be sure it is available prior to the ride.

● **HOW MUCH TO EAT**—Because everyone is unique, it is difficult to define the optimal amount of food you should eat before heading out on the bike. Studies show that most people do well with 0.5 gram of carbohydrate per pound (1 gram per kilogram) of body weight one hour before moderately hard exercise, and 2 grams of carbohydrate per pound (4 grams per kilogram) four hours beforehand (ACSM et al. 2000). For a 150-pound (70-kilogram) cyclist, this is approximately 75 to 300 grams (300 to 1,200 calories) of carbohydrates before riding—a bowl of cereal with fruit at 7 a.m. before riding at 8, to a stack of pancakes at 8 a.m. with a scheduled ride at noon.

● **EXPERIMENT DURING TRAINING**—Tolerance to pre-ride food varies greatly among riders. We know cyclists who can pile in the pancakes just before jumping on the saddle and others who can barely handle juice. What you can tolerate before (and during) a ride depends on many things, including how hard you will ride, the time of day, and your fitness level. The key to tolerating ride food is to experiment with food and drink during

You should target 0.5 grams carbohydrate (2 calories) per pound of body weight—or 1.0 gram carbohydrate (4 calories) per kilogram body weight—within an hour before you ride.

Body weight Pounds (kilograms)	Carbohydrates one hour pre-ride	
	Grams	Calories
120 (55)	60	240
140 (64)	70	280
160 (73)	80	320
180 (82)	90	360

To translate this into food, choose from the following:

Food	Carbohydrates (grams)	Calories
Bagel, 1 large	60	320
Fruit yogurt, 1 cup	50	260
Fig Newtons, 4	44	240
Spaghetti, cooked, 1 cup	40	200
Orange juice, 1 cup	25	110
Graham crackers, 4 squares	22	120
Oatmeal, cooked, 1 cup	25	150
Banana, 1 medium	25	105

1 cup = 240 milliliters

Nutrition Information from food labels, USDA National Nutrient Database (online), and J. Pennington, 2004, Bowes & Church's Food Values of Portions Commonly Used, 18th ed. (Philadelphia: Lippincott, Williams & Wilkins)

training to learn through trial and error:

- What foods and fluids work best for you, and when (do you tolerate oatmeal before a recreational ride, but only sports drink before an intense hill climb?)
- What works for you at what time of day (does your usual pre-ride bagel for afternoon rides sit like a brick for morning rides?)
- When you should consume them (do you feel best eating one hour before a ride, or three?)
- How much is appropriate (simply a banana, or a banana plus a sandwich?)

We emphasize experimenting *during training* because here is what typically happens. Cyclists read advertisements or hear fel-

❝ You'll find that individual preference for pre-ride food varies as widely as that for saddles. ❞

Bruce Ingle, Framingham, MA

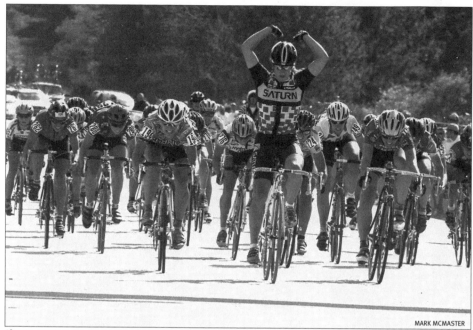

MARK MCMASTER

If you can't tolerate eating before an intense ride, plan to consume sports drinks during the ride. Experiment during training to know which brands—in which amounts—you can tolerate.

> **❝One thing I have learned is my stomach's limit! It changes for each activity I do—it's very different for swimming, biking, and running. Nothing's worse than nausea and cramps caused by overeating or eating the wrong thing! ❞**
>
> Tracie Timothy, Salt Lake City, UT

low cyclists talking about special sports drinks, energy bars, gels, supplements, or liquid meals. They may be curious about trying these products but don't get around to it...until the event day. Big mistake! In some instances they discover (much to their dismay) that the unfamiliar food or drink gives them an upset stomach, heartburn, diarrhea, or cramps, an unpleasant situation that can affect performance and morale. As one woman lamented during a racing clinic (where free samples were readily available), "This sports drink has left a terrible taste in my mouth. Does anyone have any plain water I can have?" Good thing it was only a clinic!

Realize that there will be some occasions when the tried-and-true foods that you tolerate during training may not be tolerable during a race or special ride. Chalk that up to nervousness, not the food itself.

● **TOLERATING RIDE FOOD**—Enjoying a comfortable riding experience and a good workout depend on your ability to tolerate food before and during your ride. Gastrointestinal (GI) problems are not uncommon in cycling and run the gamut from nagging heartburn and fullness to vomiting and diarrhea. Such adverse reactions occur in an estimated 30-50 percent of endurance athletes. If you are prone to GI or other food-related problems while riding, the following information can help you develop a sports nutrition plan that works best for you.

Some of the factors that can affect the ability to tolerate ride food include:

* *The intensity of exercise.* The harder you will work, the more likely you will experience GI upset. You may be able to eat within ten minutes of an easy ride, an hour before a harder ride, but need to wait three hours before a sprint or hill workout. If you exercise at a pace that you can comfortably sustain for more than 30 minutes, you can likely both exercise and digest food at the same time. At this training pace, the blood flow to your stomach is 60-70 percent of normal and is adequate to maintain normal digestion processes. During high-intensity riding, such as sprinting, racing, or hill climbing, your stomach gets about 20 percent of its normal blood flow. This slows digestion so that any pre-exercise food will simply sit along for the ride, increasing your risk for GI problems.

* *The type of exercise.* Exercise that jostles the stomach, such as running, mountain biking, or cross racing, tends to cause more stomach upset than exercise where the body bounces less, such as road cycling. Practice eating during training for the type of event you plan to do.

* *The time of exercise.* Riding at a time you are not used to riding can affect your ability to comfortably tolerate food before exercising. Your stomach may tolerate lunchtime foods before your usual afternoon ride but not breakfast foods before an unusual morning ride. If you will participate in an event that will occur at an unfa-

> **❝ For brevets that start at 3 or 4 a.m., I wake up an hour before start time, have a small amount of easy-to-digest protein (lemon yogurt works well for me), a bagel, and plenty of sports drink. If I'm starting later in the day, I have a larger breakfast three hours before departure. ❞**
> John McClellan, Groton, MA

miliar time, make sure you practice riding (and eating) at this time during training.

- *How nervous you are.* Nothing settles well when your stomach is in knots. Fuel up sufficiently the day and night before if you know you will have a case of the jitters on event day.
- *Training status.* Cyclists who are new to the sport have more GI complaints than well-trained veterans whose bodies have adapted to their riding programs. Also, experienced riders have learned what works for them during many years of riding; they have their nutrition regimen fine-tuned. If you are a novice rider, gradually increase your training volume and intensity so your body can adapt, and learn what you can and cannot handle.
- *Level of hydration.* Dehydration increases the risk of GI problems, so make sure you are well-hydrated before getting on the bike. Learn through training rides which beverages you can (and cannot) tolerate.
- *Volume of food eaten.* The stomach will take longer to empty when you eat a large meal and will leave you feeling like you are carrying a sack of bricks in your stomach during the ride. The general rule of thumb for pre-ride food is to allow:
  – 3-4 hours for a large meal to digest
  – 2-3 hours for a smaller meal
  – 1-2 hours for a blended or liquid meal
  – Less than an hour for a small snack, as tolerated

  If you want to eat a full meal before an event but fear it will upset your stomach, simply allow ample time for it to digest by eating earlier. For example, if you'll be riding at 9 a.m., plan to eat your big breakfast by 6; if you'll ride at 7 a.m. you may need to get up at 4, eat, and then go back to bed. For guidelines on eating during your ride, see chapter 9.
- *Composition of ride food.* Carbohydrates are digested more quickly than fatty foods. Low-fat meals (such as those listed in *High-Carbohydrate Meal Suggestions*, page 89) tend to digest easily and settle well. In comparison, high-fat meals such as bacon-and-egg breakfasts, cheeseburgers, tuna subs loaded with mayonnaise, and thick peanut butter sandwiches take longer to

digest, linger in the stomach, and can contribute to a weighed-down feeling, if not nausea.

A little fat, however, is appropriate. A slice of cheese on toast, some peanut butter on a bagel, or the fat in some brands of energy bars, can provide both sustained energy and satiety during long rides. Note that some cyclists can break all the sports nutrition rules and do well with even very high-fat foods. After all, steak and eggs was the Olympic breakfast of champions for many years!

- *Consistency of the food*—Liquid foods leave the stomach faster than solid foods. If a bagel before your ride or a turkey sandwich during your ride upsets your stomach, then experiment with liquids, such as juice, a smoothie, or a canned liquid meal.

> **❝ I always find time for the oatmeal-bagel-banana breakfast I routinely eat. I eat at least a half-hour before riding. I could never tolerate a greasy bacon-and-egg breakfast. ❞**
>
> **Lenny Sullivan, Methuen, MA**

● **PRE-RIDE SUGAR**—Consuming sugary carbohydrates, such as soft drinks, extra maple syrup, jellybeans, or sweetened juices just before riding, may cause hypoglycemia in sensitive individuals, leaving them fatigued, lightheaded, and shaky. If you think you may be sensitive to sugar, refer to the hypoglycemia and glycemic index information covered earlier in this chapter. Note that sugar taken during exercise generally does not contribute to a hypoglycemic reaction because muscles quickly use the sugar without the need for extra insulin. The best advice is for you to avoid the need for pre-ride sugary treats in the first place by eating appropriately timed, nourishing meals prior to exercise. If you crave sugar before an afternoon training ride, you should have eaten a bigger breakfast and lunch. Skimping on meals may leave you looking for a last-minute sugary energizer that could hurt your performance.

● SUMMARY—

- Enjoy approximately 100-300 calories of carbohydrate-rich food, as tolerated, within the hour before riding to top off your glycogen stores and enhance your stamina and energy.
- Pre-ride carbs help preserve muscle glycogen and reduce your risk of "hitting the wall"; they can also help prevent hypoglycemia, or "bonking," so you have the mental drive to finish the ride.
- In addition to offering physiological benefits, tried-and-true pre-ride foods and beverages offer a psychological value: You don't waste energy worrying about what you ate (or didn't eat).
- A number of factors affect your ability to tolerate pre-ride food, including how hard you ride, the time of day, your stress level, how hydrated you are, and kinds and amount of foods (or drinks) you consume.
- Always experiment during training to determine what pre-exercise menu works best for you to give you the most enjoyment and the best performance.

CHAPTER 9

Foods and Fluids During Long Rides

BECOMING FATIGUED IS A MAJOR CONCERN OF MOST cyclists, particularly long-distance cyclists. If you have ever "hit the wall" or "bonked," then you know how mental and physical exhaustion can slow you down, keep you from enjoying your ride, and at worst, leave you on the side of the road, waiting for the sag wagon.

You can prevent or delay the onset of fatigue during long rides by:
- preventing dehydration and
- preventing hypoglycemia (low blood sugar).

● **PREVENTING DEHYDRATION**—Sweat accounts for the majority of water lost from your body during exercise. Sweating is your body's way of dissipating heat to maintain a normal body temperature. In order to prevent dehydration during exercise you must replace sweat losses by drinking plenty of fluids.

Unfortunately by the time you may feel like drinking, you are already dehydrated and you may have lost 1 percent or more of your body weight in sweat. As you get progressively dehydrated, your breathing rate and heart rate increase, and your ability to keep from overheating decreases. The result is fatigue. Once

> ❝*With several hilly miles to go in my ride, I felt so tired and dejected; I got off the bike and nearly broke into tears. I bought a chocolate chip cookie at a nearby deli for an energy boost. It got me to the finish line! The next year, older, wiser, and better fueled, I finished three hours earlier than before—no longer the last rider.* ❞
>
> **Marilyn W., Milton, MA**

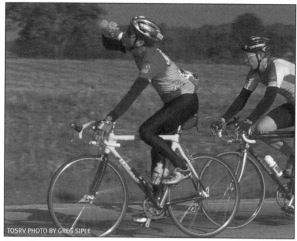

TOSRV PHOTO BY GREG SIPLE

Knowing your sweat rate helps you know how much to drink during your rides. Consume at least 16 ounces (480 milliliters) of fluid for every pound (.45 kilograms) of sweat you lose.

dehydrated during exercise, you'll have a very hard time correcting the imbalance.

Since your body's thirst mechanism is not a reliable signal to drink, plan to drink on a schedule before you feel thirsty. As a general rule, drink 8 ounces (240 milliliters), roughly 8 gulps, of water or sports drink every 15 to 20 minutes during hot and sweaty exercise. This is far less than what most cyclists would voluntarily consume.

To be safe, you should know your sweat rate and fluid targets (see chapter 7) and practice meeting your fluid goals during training. If you are not used to consuming this much fluid while biking, you can train your gut to handle this volume by gradually increasing your fluid intake during training rides. Marking your water bottles in 8-ounce (240-milliliter) increments or setting your watch or bike computer to remind you to drink at regular intervals can be helpful.

Do not drink more water than you can handle. The immediate solution to "stomach sloshing" is to stop drinking for a while. The long-term solution is to practice drinking during training, so your body can adapt to the appropriate fluid intake.

Here are a few tips on how to prevent dehydration.

• *Take advantage of every opportunity to drink.* If you are participating in a supported ride, take advantage of every checkpoint or stop along the route by drinking from and then topping-off your water bottles. (But do not over-hydrate.)

- *Bring your own fluids for competitive events.* If you are in a race, bring enough of your own preferred fluid. Don't rely on race promoters to have water or your favorite sports drink available. While racing, gulp from your bottle at every opportunity, and don't get so caught up in the excitement that you forget to drink and fall short of your fluid goals.

- *Plan water stops or bring a ride's supply.* For unsupported rides, select a route that includes water fountains, convenience stores, or cafes. If you are riding in a remote location, take with you all the fluids that you will need for the ride. Some cyclists use a Camelbak (water reservoir that straps to your back) or another portable hydration system, which offers the advantage of high volume—the larger ones can hold up to 100 ounces (12.5 cups or 2.8 liters) of fluid, enough for several hours of cycling. If you prefer to use water bottles, you can load multiple bottle cages on the bike (on the frame, behind the seat, on the handlebars) or carry extra filled bottles in jersey pockets or a pannier.

- *Become proficient at drinking while riding.* Practice your bike-handling skills every time you ride: drinking while pedaling, climbing, braking, or riding in a pack; drinking with either hand; switching water bottles from front cage to back; and retrieving water bottles out of your jersey pockets. The more comfortable you feel doing these things, the more likely you are to drink as frequently as you should, and the safer you are on the bike doing so.

For more information on fluids, water, and hydration, see chapter 7.

- **PREVENTING HYPOGLYCEMIA**—Because your brain controls your muscles and your ability to concentrate on the task at hand, you'll ride better if your brain is well-fed. The brain relies on blood sugar for fuel. When you experience hypoglycemia (low blood sugar), you will feel lightheaded, dizzy, irritable, very tired—and

❝It's good to keep five bucks in your pocket so you can buy something to get you home if you bonk. Any quick sugar—a can of Coke or juice—can do the trick to get blood sugar back up. Otherwise, you will be ready to stick your thumb out and hitch a ride home! ❞

Adam Hodges Myerson
Northampton, MA

question if you are able to go on riding. Your judgment and decision-making may be impaired, which can cost you the race or cause you to ride unsafely. Most athletes describe this condition as "bonking."

To prevent hypoglycemia, you need to fuel up before the ride (see chapter 8) and consume carbohydrates during the ride. You can significantly improve your stamina by consuming 100 to 250 calories (25 to 60 grams) of carbohydrates per hour of cycling after the first hour (ACSM 2000), depending on your body size and ability to tolerate fuel while you bike. This may be:

- 4 cups (1 liter) of a sports drink (200 calories)
- 16 ounces (0.5 liters) of sports drink (100 calories) + a banana or half of a sports bar (100 calories) + extra water
- 4 fig cookies (250 calories) + extra water

This may be too few calories for some cyclists and it may be more calories than other cyclists voluntarily consume during a long ride.

Practice consuming a variety of solid or liquid carbohydrates—juice, gels, dried fruit, granola bars, lemonade, energy bars, jellybeans, whatever. Very fast riders and elite racers tend to prefer sports drinks or gels. Slower riders who don't hammer through their ride can thrive with a variety of regular foods and fluids. Despite popular belief, even refined sugar (like jellybeans, sugar cubes, and soft drinks) can be a positive snack while cycling.

Many cyclists fear that fluids or foods taken during a ride or race will cause diarrhea. Generally, this is not true. Diarrhea commonly occurs in *dehydrated* cyclists who have lost more than 4 percent of their body weight. Drinking fluids can help prevent diarrhea, not cause it.

Experiment for yourself during training and devise a program for eating and drinking for riding so you know what, when, and how much you like to consume for the best perfor-

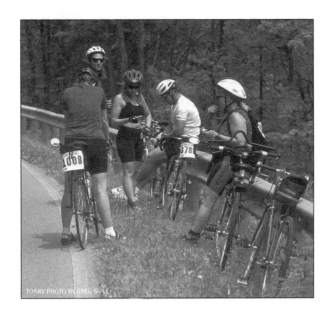
TOSRV PHOTO BY GREG SIPLE

66On long training rides I used to carry bananas, bagels, and Fig Newtons in my jersey pockets. I've replaced much of this stuff with carbohydrate gels— they are easier to carry, though not quite as tasty or nutritious. I always keep one or two stashed in my saddle bag for emergency fuel. 99

Bill O'Mara, Andover, MA

mance. Refer to page 98, *Popular Foods and Fluids During Long Rides*.

Here are a few tips to help you prevent hypoglycemia:

- *Bring carbohydrates with you.* Jerseys or jackets with multiple, easy-to-reach pockets are a good way to carry your snacks. You can grab the food while riding and avoid the need to stop to eat. If you prefer to drink your carbohydrates, bring enough sports drink or other liquid carbohydrate for the ride. For longer distances, consider bringing powered sports drink to which you simply add water.

- *Replenish your supplies along the way.* For long events, you might want to have friends replenish your supplies by meeting you at designated areas along the course. Or, plan a route that has stores where you can buy food and beverages.

- *Make a plan.* For stressful events, think ahead and make a clear plan before the event day. Plan what, when, and how you will eat and drink, and make sure you have practiced this in training. This is especially important for less seasoned riders or for those doing their first event. You must also be flexible—who knows what you will tolerate when your body and mind are pushed to the limit! Even tried-and-true favorites can become unpalatable.

- *Know what foods and fluids you tolerate.* To avoid unwanted surprises such as heartburn, diarrhea, or upset stomach during an event, avoid foods or sports drinks that you have not tried during training. Your training rides are the time to sample unfamiliar food and drink.

- *Choose either solid or liquid carbohydrates.* Many cyclists prefer to drink their carbohydrates in the form of sugary fluid such as a sports drink, diluted juice or defizzed cola. But solid foods can work well, too, as long as you drink plenty of water and can tolerate the food.

- *Become proficient at eating while riding.* Practice your bike-handling/eating skills every time you ride. Practice getting food out of your jersey pocket, unwrapping it, and eating it, while pedaling, coasting, or riding in a pack. If you're right-handed, keep food in the left pocket and reach back with the left hand so that your strongest hand/arm stays connected to the handlebar (or do the opposite if you are left-handed). The more comfortable you are eating on the bike, the safer you'll be and the more likely you are to eat as much as you should.

- *Prepare and stash your bike food so it's easily accessible.* During training find out what foods are the best for you to carry, open, and eat while riding. Experiment with small plastic bags to learn which ones are easiest to handle. Before the ride, unwrap or tear open energy bars so you don't have to fuss with wrappers while riding. Portion your hourly food into separate small bags (and consume the contents of one bag per hour). Figure out what food to stash in your back or front jersey pocket for

easy access, and what to tuck away in your bike bag or pannier. Some cyclists tape gel packets or energy bars to their handlebars; others put unwrapped food directly in their (clean) jersey pockets! Remember where you put your food and pack it the same way each time so that eating becomes a habit.

- *To save room and weight, carry powdered beverages or sports drinks.* This only applies if you will have access to water to reconstitute them.

- **SPORTS FOODS AND DRINKS**—There is no magic to the special sports bars, gels, or drinks that are marketed to cyclists. These engineered products offer no nutritional advantage over regular food or drink. What they do offer is convenience in a pre-wrapped, easy, and portable package. Whichever way you choose to consume your fuel is fine as long as it works for you.

Some people find they tolerate commercial sports drinks better than other carbohydrate fluids such as juice or soft drinks. Sports drinks are dilute solutions of carbohydrates with a few electrolytes added to aid in absorption. They contain much less carbohydrate per ounce than highly concentrated carbohydrate fluids like juice and soft drinks (and solid food, for that matter).

You can dilute ordinary beverages with water (such as a 1:1 ratio of orange juice and water) and add a dash of salt to create a carbohydrate drink with a profile similar to a commercial sports drink. To make your own sports drink, see the recipe on page 76.

Beware that while they may be fortified, commercial sports foods and drinks lack many of the vitamins and minerals, antioxidants, fiber and other nutrients that natural foods contain. They also tend to be more expensive than standard foods. The bottom line is choose a carbohydrate food or drink that you like and that you know you tolerate.

- **FOOD TOLERANCE**—Fear of stomach upset can deter some riders from eating during rides. On the other hand, fear of bonking or hitting the wall can lead other riders to overeat during rides, leading to stomach upset. Through trial and error during training rides, you can find what works for you. Refer back to the previous chapter to *Tolerating*

> *For cool-weather, long-ride days, I carry baggies of Carnation Instant Breakfast mix with two heaping tablespoons of powdered milk, a tablespoon of sugar, and cocoa powder. I make several baggies—one bag equals one bottle. To reconstitute at water stops, I empty the contents into a tall water bottle, add cold water and shake. It's substantial nourishment (enough for one hour for me), and it tastes like a chocolate milkshake.*
>
> Jenny Hegmann, Reading, MA

You should target at least 100 to 250 calories (25 to 60 grams) of carbohydrates and about 24 to 32 ounces (750 milliliters to 1000 milliliters) of fluid per hour while on the bike. Here is a listing of some popular biking foods and fluids.

Foods	Amount	Calories	Carb. (grams)	Protein (grams)	Fat (grams)
Almonds/peanuts	1 oz.	160	7	4	15
Bagel, plain	1 medium	250	47	9	1
Banana	1 medium	105	26	1	0
Cheese, reduced-fat	1 oz.	80	0	7	6
Dates, dried	5	120	30	0	0
Fig Newtons	1	60	11	1	1
Go-Gurt (yogurt in a tube)	2.25 oz.	80	13	2	2
Granola bar, plain, hard	1 bar (1 oz.)	130	18	3	5
Kellogs PopTart (blueberry frosted)	1	210	37	2	6
Oatmeal cookie	1 medium	65	10	1	2
Orange	1 medium	70	17	1	0
Peanut butter and jelly sandwich	1 small	360	45	14	16
York Peppermint Patty	1.5 oz.	165	35	1	3
Raisins	1/3 cup	160	40	2	0
Snickers candy bar	2.16-oz.	280	37	6	14

1/3 cup = 80 milliliters; 1 tablespoon = 15 milliliters; 1 ounce = 28 grams; 4 ounces = 120 milliliters

Nutrition information from food labels and J. Pennington, 2004, Bowes & Church's Food Values of Portions Commonly Used, 18th ed. (Philadelphia: Lippincott, Williams & Wilkins).

❝For long rides, chocolate milk is a terrific way to get both fluids and a pile of calories in real fast! It's always available at convenience stores in 16-ounce containers. ❞

Ed Kross, Framingham, MA

Ride Food on page 87, to learn some tips about food before and during exercise.

Endurance cyclists, touring cyclists, and randonneurs who are on the bike for long hours and often days at a stretch, can suffer from taste fatigue especially if they are using only commercial sports foods. Sweet, high-carbohydrate foods and fluids all day long can become monotonous. During your training, try a variety of standard foods and fluids, like sandwiches, thick-crust pizza, and pretzels, to see what you tolerate. This way, if you begin to crave a hamburger in your 80th mile (or 8th hour or 8th day) you'll know whether you can (or cannot) handle one.

Foods	Amount	Calories	Carb. (grams)	Protein (grams)	Fat (grams)
Beverages					
Carnation Instant Breakfast	1 packet	130	25	6	0
Cranberry juice cocktail	8 oz.	145	36	0	0
Defizzed cola	12 oz.	160	40	0	0
Chocolate low-fat milk	8 oz.	155	26	8	2
Orange juice	8 oz.	110	26	2	0
Energy Bars/Gels					
Clif	1 bar	240	45	10	4.5
Extran Endurance Bar	1 bar	225	50	1	2
Luna	1 bar	180	27	10	4
PowerBar Harvest	1 bar	240	45	7	4.5
PowerBar Performance	1 bar	230	45	10	2.5
SmartFuel Warpbar	1 bar	180	31	8	3.5
Gu	1 packet	100	25	0	0
Hammer Gel	2 tablespoons	90	23	0	0
Powdered Sports Drinks/Per 25 to 30 grams					
Accelerade	1 scoop	120	21	5	1
Cytomax	1 scoop	95	20	0	0
Extran Thirst Quencher	1 scoop	30	7	0	0
Gatorade	1¹/₃ scoop	120	30	0	0
Hammer Sustained Energy	1 scoop	110	24	3	0
SmartFuel WarpAide	³/₄ scoop	110	27	0	0

• **FAT DURING EXERCISE**—While carbohydrates are an important fuel during exercise, you need not eat only carbs. Eating a little fat is okay, too. Fat-containing foods provide sustained energy. A little fat—such as that in a peanut butter sandwich, cheese on a roll, granola bar, cookie, or energy bar—helps food digest more slowly and therefore can provide longer lasting energy for people who will be riding for more than a couple hours.

• **PROTEIN DURING EXERCISE**—During endurance exercise, your body breaks down a little of its muscle protein. Consuming some protein before, during, and after exercise can help to offset this

> **❝On a longer ride, I'll routinely have fruit, a turkey sandwich, and pretzels. The chili always smells oh-so-good, but I avoid it because I'm not sure how it will affect me on the ride. ❞**
>
> John Polakas, Brooklyn, NY

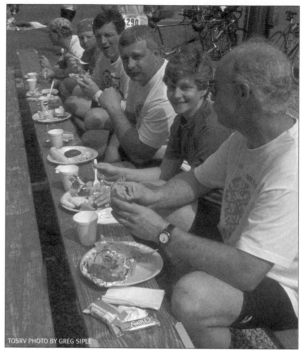

TOSRV PHOTO BY GREG SIPLE

By experimenting with your food and drink during training, you can minimize stomach upset during long rides and special events.

loss and improve protein balance (Koopman et al. 2004). Some popular protein foods include an egg or milk with the pre-ride breakfast, chocolate milk or a few nuts during the ride, and turkey (in a sandwich) after the ride. Many sports drinks and bars are are now fortified with protein. Of course, protein should never up-stage carbohydrates as your primary fuel for cycling.

● **SUMMARY**—All too often riders hold off until after their ride to enjoy a good meal. They end up needlessly fatigued and overly hungry. Why wait until after your ride to enjoy the fuel that could have enhanced your performance and enjoyment during the ride?

● The fluids and foods that you consume during your rides should be an extension of your carbohydrate-rich daily training diet.

- Preventing dehydration and low blood sugar (hypoglycemia) are the keys to preventing fatigue.
- To prevent dehydration, know your sweat rate and replace fluids accordingly. Drink on a regular schedule, targeting about 8 ounces (240 milliliters) of fluid every 15 to 20 minutes.
- To prevent hypoglycemia, target at least 100 to 250 calories from carbohydrates during each hour of your ride.
- Sports foods, gels, and drinks while easy and convenient, can be costly and offer no better nutrition than standard foods. They lack many of the nutrients that real food provides.
- Learn through trial and error during training what foods and fluids settle best and contribute to top performance.
- During training you should: develop a feeding and fluid plan for the event; learn your fluid targets and your calorie targets and the foods and fluids you will need to achieve these targets; and know how you will access your foods and fluids during your event.

❝ For an endurance ride, I eat a peanut-butter-and-honey sandwich, baked chips (for salt), and the occasional cookie. For me, these foods work better than energy bars, and they're a fraction of the cost. ❞

Marilyn W., Milton, MA

CHAPTER 10

Recovering from Exhaustive Rides

JUST AS FUELING BEFORE AND DURING RIDING IS IMPORTANT, SO IS refueling afterwards. Your post-ride sports diet is critical to full and speedy recovery—to replenish depleted glycogen stores, help heal damaged muscles, rehydrate body tissues, and restore electrolytes—which allows you to endure repeated days (and weeks) of hard training, racing, or touring. Poor recovery practices take their toll, limiting how hard you can train, how fast you can improve, and how good you feel on and off the bike. The most important considerations for recovery are fluids and carbohydrates, as well as when you consume them after exercise.

> **"After riding hard, I usually spin down for 10 to 20 minutes, then stretch. I make sure to drink some kind of recovery drink immediately and eat within 30 minutes. I also make sure to drink lots of fluids. "**
>
> Jessica Truslow, Arlington, MA

● **RECOVERY FLUIDS**—Your first priority after a hard ride should be to replace fluid losses as soon as possible. Ideally, you should have minimized dehydration by drinking plenty of fluids and replacing sweat losses on schedule while riding (see chapter 7). Here are answers to some of the questions you may have about rehydration:

When and how much should I drink after I ride?—As soon as you get off the bike, drink enough to quench your thirst, and then drink more. You might not feel thirsty immediately nor for several hours, but your body may still need fluid. Your goal is to have pale-colored urine in significant quantity, a sign that you are appropriately hydrated.

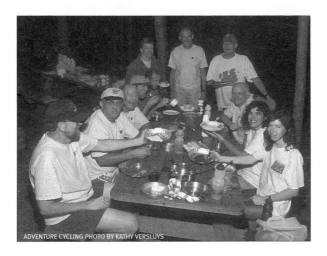

Sharing enjoyable recovery meals with riding companions adds to your cycling memories.

---

66 *We rode from Alaska to Argentina. There were days we felt we couldn't eat enough. One night we ate three dinners. In Peru, we walked into town and had a good dinner. Afterward, we passed another restaurant, could smell chicken roasting, and enjoyed a second dinner. Our third dinner was provided by our generous (and unsuspecting) hosts. Those were wonderful days when we were able to eat constantly and convert those calories to miles and miles.* **99**

Greg and June Siple, Missoula, MT

Make sure recovery fluids will be available at the end of your ride, wherever that will be. Plan to end your ride at a home or a convenience store, or pack your favorite recovery fluids with you in an ice-filled cooler to take along in the car. It is also a good idea to keep a gallon of water in your car so you will have fluid available when you or your thirsty companions need it.

What's best to drink? Are sports drinks preferable?—Good fluid choices include any that taste good to you, so you'll drink plenty of them: water, juices, sports drinks, soft drinks, lemonade, sweetened ice tea, or whatever you prefer. Here is information on some popular fluids to help you choose what is best for you:

- *Water.* Plain water provides fluid but not the carbohydrates you need to replenish depleted muscle glycogen. Thus, you should eat carbohydrate-rich foods with the water, such as a bagel, fruit, or energy bar. Because sodium enhances fluid absorption and retention, eat some salty foods with your water, such as pretzels or salted nuts, especially if you were biking in hot weather and have lost a lot of sweat.
- *Soft drinks.* Although they lack nutritional value and are filled with empty calories, soft drinks offer both carbohydrates and

fluids. Cola offers caffeine, which for some may provide welcome stimulation. Historically, athletes have been told to avoid caffeine, believed to be a diuretic that would hamper efforts to replace fluids. But now we know that caffeine has no diuretic effect in athletes who are accustomed to consuming it and is not likely to hurt recovery (Armstrong 2002). Because soft drinks lack sodium, also consume some salty foods.

- *Juices.* Fruit and vegetable juices are excellent choices because they are carbohydrate-rich and they offer the vitamin C your body needs to optimize healing. Salty vegetable juices, such as V8 or tomato juice, aid in fluid absorption and retention. Fruit juice, like water and soft drinks, lacks sodium, so consume some salty foods with your fruit juice. Or put a pinch of salt into each 8-ounce (240-milliliter) cup of juice, giving you roughly 85 milligrams of sodium per cup, comparable to many sports drinks.

- *Sports drinks.* Commercial fluid replacers designed to be taken during exercise (such as Gatorade) are dilute solutions of sugar in water with a small amount of sodium added. You will get many more carbohydrates per ounce by drinking juice. For example, you would have to drink 48 ounces (1.3 liters) of commercial fluid replacer to get the carbohydrates contained in just 16 ounces (480 milliliters) of cranberry-apple juice. If you choose fruit juice, remember to also have a salty snack.

- *Commercial recovery drinks.* These high-carbohydrate beverages are sweetened with a type of sugar that tastes less sweet so it is more palatable in high concentrations. Some recovery drinks contain small amounts of protein, which may help enhance glycogen synthesis and muscle repair. However, research is conflicting (see the section on recovery protein on page 108). You can achieve your protein needs without such recovery drinks by enjoying some protein-containing foods as part of your recovery plan (such as sweetened yogurt with crackers, cheese or salted peanuts with fruit juice, chocolate milk with pretzels), and also by eating adequate protein on a daily basis. Commercial recov-

❝I only drink wine or beer if I know I am not riding the next day. If I am dehydrated after a long ride, alcohol puts me in a deeper hole in terms of recovery. Riding is not fun when you are dehydrated! ❞

Jessica Truslow, Arlington, MA

ery drinks are convenient, if costly, but they offer nothing that cannot be found in standard foods.

Is beer a good recovery fluid?—Beer is often a part of post-ride festivities. But when you are dehydrated and hungry, drinking alcohol on an empty stomach can hit you like a ton of bricks. Like wine and other spirits, beer lacks the carbohydrates you need to replenish your glycogen stores—a 12-ounce bottle has just 11 to 13 grams of carbohydrates, fewer carbs than a slice of bread. Drinking alcohol post-ride impairs glycogen synthesis by displacing carbohydrates from your recovery diet (Burke et al. 2003). If you plan to consume alcohol as part of your recovery meal, first drink plenty of other fluids and eat some salty, high-carbohydrate foods. Then, continue to sip water (or juice or soft drinks) and nibble on recovery foods while you enjoy your beer: rolls, baked potato with salt, crackers, or thick-crust pizza.

For more on recovery fluids, see *Comparing Fluid Replacers* in chapter 7.

● **RECOVERY CARBOHYDRATES**—After rehydrating, your next priority after a ride should be replenishing your glycogen (carbohydrate) stores. Eat carbohydrate-rich foods beginning as soon as possible after exercise and continue for several hours for the fastest and most complete restoration of glycogen in depleted muscles. Cyclists who fail to recover with adequate carbohydrates will lack the fuel and energy to ride strongly the next day. This is a particular concern for long-distance touring cyclists, racers, and or those who train hard every day (or twice a day).

In addition to recovery carbohydrates, you should eat a daily diet that is carbohydrate-based, with abundant grains and cereals, starchy vegetables (peas, potatoes), fruits, and legumes (dried beans and peas, lentils, hummus). As a guideline, carbohydrate foods such as these should take up half to three-quarters of the space on your plate. This will help you to

> **"When touring, one of our favorite dinners was breakfast: pancakes, eggs, ham, and fruit salad. Apart from the occasional rest day, we never took time for a cooked breakfast, so this was a treat— carbohydrate-rich, balanced with protein, and perfect for refueling our tired muscles. "**
>
> Candace Crowell, Georgetown, MA

To facilitate speedy recovery, drink fluids and consume carbohydrates as soon as possible after riding.

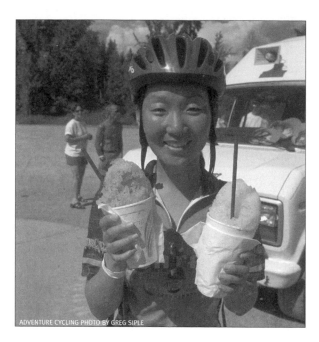

ADVENTURE CYCLING PHOTO BY GREG SIPLE

> **❝I make a really big bowl of tri-colored pasta and chicken the day before a century ride to enjoy for recovery afterward. ❞**
>
> Steve Chabra, New York, NY

> **❝I drink a glass of juice or chocolate milk (or whatever high-carb drink is in the fridge) within 10 minutes of walking in the house from a hard or long ride. I'll also grab something salty—a handful of salty baked chips, sunflower seeds or pretzel sticks— because I'm craving salt. I've noticed a direct correlation: eat sooner, recover sooner...feel better, ride better! ❞**
>
> Louise Wilcox, Reading, MA

avoid the gradual and chronic glycogen depletion that can occur with repeated days and weeks of hard riding. Here are answers to some of the questions cyclists often ask about carbs.

When should I eat after my rides?—As soon as possible after hard exercise, you should begin replenishing your glycogen stores by consuming carbohydrates. We say as soon as possible because immediately following hard exercise, the enzymes responsible for making glycogen are most active and will most rapidly replace depleted glycogen stores. The most rapid glycogen synthesis occurs within 60 to 90 minutes following hard exercise. This is particularly important for riders who train hard on repeated days or who train more than once a day. Glycogen stores can be completely restored within 24 hours or sooner if the intake and timing of carbohydrate is right.

How many carbohydrates do I need to recover?—For optimal glycogen recovery, you should consume 0.5 gram of carbohydrate per pound (1.0 gram per kilogram) of body weight each hour after getting off the bike until you are able to sit down to a regular meal. A 150-pound (70-kilogram) cyclist needs approximately 75 grams (300 calories) of carbohydrates per hour for several hours after exercise. It is best to consume the carbohydrates in 30-minute intervals (Ivy 2001). You can accomplish this by nibbling on snacks or by sipping on carbohydrate-containing beverages. For example, drink 8 ounces (240 milliliters) of cranberry juice (40 grams of carbohydrate) the minute you end your ride and then 30 minutes later have another 8 ounces of cranberry juice.

Note it's the amount of carbohydrate not the calories that is important for recovery. You should consume 75 grams (300 calories) of carbohydrates, not just 300 calories of anything (if you weigh 150 pounds or 70 kilograms). For example, an energy bar has close to 300 calories, but it may have far less than 75 grams of carbohydrates. In this case, you should eat two energy bars or drink enough orange juice with the bar to meet your carbohydrate goal. If you eat a 300-calorie sandwich (such a turkey or peanut butter sandwich), you likely are getting only 30 to 40 grams of carbohydrates, so be sure to also drink juice, put extra jelly on the peanut butter, or have a few plain cookies.

> **❝I buy bananas, peel them, cut them into chunks, and keep them frozen so I can blend them with milk and juice for a recovery shake after riding. ❞**
>
> Paul Humphries, Reading, MA

What are the best recovery carbs?—Although all carbohydrates will help to replenish your depleted glycogen stores, easily digestible, moderate to high glycemic carbohydrates should be the major carbohydrate choice in recovery meals (Burke et al. 2004). This is because the more easily the food is digested, the faster it is converted to glucose in the blood and the quicker your muscles have the substrate they need for making glycogen. High glycemic index foods include bagels, potatoes, many breakfast cereals, sports drinks, and honey, just to name a few. You can check the glycemic index of more foods on page 81.

If exercise kills your appetite or if even the thought of post-exercise food makes you nauseated, you can drink the carbohydrates (and simultaneously provide your body with the fluid it needs to recover). This is why blenderized drinks, or fruit-

● RECOMMENDED CARBOHYDRATE INTAKE FOR RECOVERY

Your muscles are most receptive to replacing depleted glycogen stores immediately after exercise. For optimal recovery, consume approximately 0.5 gram of carbohydrate per pound (1.0 gram per kilogram) of body weight each hour following exercise until your regular eating pattern can be resumed. You should also include a little protein for muscle recovery. (Sodium and potassium are also important recovery nutrients. See the charts on pages 112-113.)

Carbohydrates for recovery per hour after exercise:

| Body weight | | Carbohydrate | Body weight | | Carbohydrate |
lbs	(kg)	grams	lbs	(kg)	grams
120	(55)	60	170	(77)	85
130	60)	65	180	(82)	90
140	(64)	70	190	(86)	95
150	(70)	75	200	(90)	100
160	(73)	80	210	(95)	105

and-milk "smoothies," and juices are popular choices for many cyclists. With time, your hunger will return. For some people, this may not be until the next day.

Will eating protein with the carbs help me recover faster?—Maybe. Some researchers believe that eating a small amount of protein along with recovery carbohydrates (such as milk with cereal, meat on bread, yogurt with juice) may improve the body's protein balance (Koopman 2004), or enhance glycogen synthesis and muscle repair (Ivy et al. 2002, Ivy 2001). Other research suggests eating protein does not significantly improve the rate of muscle glycogen synthesis when adequate carbohydrates are consumed following exercise (Jentjens et al. 2001, Zachweija 2002), but that it may reduce muscle soreness (Flakoll et al. 2004). For more on protein refer to chapter 5 and see page 104. Eating some protein as part of your recovery food plan is recommended as long as it does not interfere with your consuming adequate carbohydrates. In other words, don't fill up on the post-ride barbecued chicken and overlook the bread, potato, or pasta!

● **RECOVERY ELECTROLYTES**—Here are answers to commonly asked questions about electrolyte replacement after riding

Here is the carbohydrate and protein content of some selected recovery fluids and foods. Please refer to the table on page 98 in the previous chapter for more items.

Fluids	Amount	Calories	Carb. (g)	Protein (g)
Grapefruit juice	1 cup	95	22	0
V8 Juice	1 cup	50	10	0
Soymilk	1 cup	120	12	10
Lemonade	16 oz.	150	35	0
Chocolate low-fat milk	1 cup	155	26	8
Foods				
Baked potato or sweet potato w/skin	1 large	280	60	7
Chicken-rice or lentil soup	1 cup	130	20	9
Baked beans	1 cup	235	50	15
Fruit yogurt (low-fat)	8 ounces	225	40	8
Frozen yogurt (low-fat)	1 cup	230	35	6
Jelly, jam, honey, maple syrup, or sugar	1 tablespoon	50	13	0
Bagel	1 large	330	65	12
White or whole-wheat bread	1 slice	65-90	15-20	2-4
Cornflakes with 4 oz. milk	1 cup cereal	150	35	7
Oatmeal, cooked	1 cup	145	25	6
Rice, boiled	1 cup	265	55	5
Pretzels	1 oz.	110	25	2
Peanut butter and jelly sandwich	1 sandwich	360	45	14
Hamburger (McDonald's)	1 small	280	35	13
Cheese pizza (12-inch)	¹/₂ pie	560	80	25
Bean burrito without cheese (Taco Bell)	1 small	300	55	10
Spaghetti with tomato sauce	1¹/₂ cups	230	45	9
Turkey sub (Subway)	6-inch	280	45	18
Commercial Recovery Drinks				
Endurox R4	2 scoops	270	52	13
Smartfuel BioFix	2 scoops	290	60	11
Cytomax Recovery	2 scoops	350	18	26
Hammer Recoverite	2 scoops	166	32	10

Nutrition information from food labels, product websites, USDA National Nutrient Database (online), and J. Pennington, 2004, Bowes & Church's Food Values of Portions Commonly Used, 18th ed. (Philadelphia: Lippincott, Williams & Wilkins)

1 cup = 240 milliliters; 1 tablespoon = 15 milliliters; 1 ounce = 28 grams

Do I need extra salt to replace what I lose in sweat?—Cyclists lose some sodium in sweat but are unlikely to deplete their body stores during typical cycling events that last under four to six hours. In most cases, cyclists and other endurance athletes can replace more than enough sodium by eating everyday foods that contain sodium during and after exercise.

Sodium is found in foods naturally and is also a part of salt. Each teaspoon (5 grams) of salt contains 2,300 milligrams of sodium. During three hours of sweaty exercise, you might lose 1,200 to 4,500 milligrams of sodium. Since the average 150-pound (70-kilogram) body contains about 75,000 milligrams of sodium, this 2 to 6 percent loss is relatively insignificant. See chapter 7 for more on salt and sodium.

Cyclists who may need *extra* salt include those who ride in the heat the entire day, tour in hot weather for multiple days, or train in cold weather yet do their event (race, tour, etc.) in warm weather. To get extra salt, you do not need salt tablets. Consuming regular foods that contain salt gives you plenty of sodium: pasta with tomato sauce, pizza, deli turkey slices, tomato or V8 juice, salad dressings, pickles, salted nuts. Check food labels and you may be surprised at the sodium content of many everyday foods. If you crave salt, you should respond appropriately by eating sodium-rich foods that are also rich in carbohydrates, such as baked potatoes with salt or ketchup, salted pretzels, and soups.

Do I need extra potassium?—Like sodium, you lose some potassium when you sweat, but you are unlikely to deplete your body stores. During three hours of sweaty exercise, you might lose 300 to 1,200 milligrams of potassium (.001 to .007 percent of your body stores). The typical American diet provides 4,000 to 7,000 milligrams of potassium each day and easily replaces that lost in sweat, particularly if you eat potassium-rich foods, such as fruits and vegetables. On pages 112-113 is a list of popular recovery foods and their sodium and potassium content. Some of these foods also work well during long rides (see chapter 9).

● **RECOVERY PROTEIN**—In addition to fluids, carbohydrates, and electrolytes, protein is also important for recovery.

Do I need extra protein?—Adequate protein is necessary to repair and rebuild muscles damaged by hard exercise. But you do not need to eat a high-protein diet. If you eat too much meat and other protein foods, you'll choose less of the carbohydrate-rich foods needed to refuel depleted glycogen stores.

Cyclists can consume their protein needs by eating a balanced training diet. If you eat a serving of protein-rich food at two meals (such as a turkey sandwich at lunch and spaghetti with meat sauce for a recovery dinner) and consume three servings of low-fat dairy foods (such as yogurt with breakfast, low-fat cheese on sandwich at lunch, and chocolate low-fat milk for a post-ride recovery snack) each day, you'll provide your body with enough protein to build and repair muscles. Refer to chapter 5 for more on protein.

Consuming some protein along with your recovery carbohydrates may enhance recovery. Refer to page 108.

What are good sources of protein for recovery?—Many cyclists report craving protein, particularly red meat, after hard exercise. If that is the case for you, eat the protein and be sure to eat carbohydrate-rich foods with it. Enjoy a large potato and rolls with your steak; a bagel with eggs; hearty bread with peanut butter; or a bowl of rice or pasta with chicken or fish. This balance will help you rebuild and refuel, as well as enjoy the process.

Vegetarian cyclists can meet their protein requirements by carefully choosing plenty of non-animal sources of protein, such as soymilk, tofu, tempeh, beans, peas, and lentils. These foods have the advantage of offering not only

> **" My favorite recovery foods are salted, dry roasted peanuts and a stack of Fig Newtons. "**
> Earl Fernstermacher, Seattle, WA

> **" After a very long event, I'm usually craving protein, so the hamburger stops being a fantasy and becomes a reality. "**
> John McClellan, Groton, MA

During two hours of moderately sweaty riding, you might lose 400 milligrams of potassium and 3,000 milligrams of sodium in your sweat. To replace these electrolytes you can include some of these popular foods in your recovery plan. (Also see *Comparing Fluid Replacers* on page 71 in chapter 7.)

Sodium: Rich sources include any food processed with salt, such as canned vegetable products, baked goods, and fast foods (choose fast foods carefully, as they can also be rich sources of fat).

Food	Amount	Sodium (mg)
Canned soup or baked beans	1 cup	1,010
Deli ham, turkey, or roast beef	3 ounces	750-1,200
Cheese pizza	¹/₄ of 12-inch pie	700
V8 juice	8 ounces	740
Spaghetti sauce	¹/₂ cup	600
Salt	¹/₄ teaspoon	575
Bagel	1 medium	550
Hamburger (McDonald's)	1 small	550
Muffin	1 medium	500
Salted pretzels	1 ounce	485
Saltine crackers	10	400
Ketchup	2 tablespoons	360

> **"In racing season we have a training ride every Wednesday night. It's a tradition that we meet at the local burrito place after the ride—I get a burrito with rice, black beans, potatoes, and carrots."**
>
> Adam Hodges Myerson,
> Northampton, MA

protein but also carbohydrate, which meat, fish, eggs, and poultry lack. Some energy bars contain soy protein, as well. For more on vegetarian diets see chapter 5.

● **RECOVERY AND WEIGHT LOSS**—If you are trying to lose weight, recovery time is not the time to do it. Some weight-conscious cyclists use the time during and after a ride to diet and try to lose weight. They figure that by restricting food, they will not be replacing "all the calories" that they have burned during the ride. Yes, it is true that you will burn body fat by restricting calories before, during, or after a ride, but you will also lack energy to ride strongly, enjoy riding, and recover your

Potassium: *Excellent sources include fruits, juices, vegetables, and dairy products.*

Food	Amount	Potassium (mg)
Potato, sweet or white, baked	1 large	715-845
Baked beans	1 cup	750
V8 juice	1 cup	510
Cantaloupe	1/4 melon	500
Orange juice	1 cup	475
Banana	1 medium	450
Milk, chocolate low-fat	1 cup	425
Vegetable soup	1 cup	395
Milk, low-fat	1 cup	380
Fruit yogurt	1 cup	450
Raisins	1/4 cup	300

Note: sports drinks are generally poor sources of both potassium and sodium:

Per 8 ounces	Potassium (mg)	Sodium (mg)
Gatorade	30	110
Accelerade	40	125
Cytomax	80	75
Powerade	30	55

1 cup = 240 milliliters; 1 tablespoon = 15 milliliters; 1 ounce = 28 grams; 1/4 teaspoon = 1 gram

Nutrition information from food labels, USDA National Nutrient Database (online), and J. Pennington, 2004, Bowes & Church's Food Values of Portions Commonly Used, 18th ed. (Philadelphia: Lippincott, Williams & Wilkins)

tired muscles for tomorrow's ride. In addition to needless fatigue, denying yourself adequate nourishment for riding and recovery can lead to extreme hunger, carbohydrate cravings, and out-of-control food binges that contribute to weight gain.

Your best bet for reducing body fat is to fuel appropriately for riding by consuming adequate carbohydrates before, during, and after riding. Then cut back on calories, particularly calories from fat and alcohol, after you have fully recovered, for instance, on rest days or later in the evening. Your goal is to have energy during the day for cycling; you can then eat less at night and on rest days when your body requires less fuel. Ideally, you should try to shed extra body fat during the off-season or early-season training when you are not putting such physical demands on your body. For more on weight and reduction of body fat see chapter 14.

The optimal refueling plan includes plenty of carbohydrates to restore glycogen, some protein to help heal damaged muscles, and sodium and potassium to replace that lost in sweat. If circumstances prevent you from sitting down to a recovery meal (or if you have no appetite) for several hours after your ride, you should consume enough carbohydrates immediately following your ride by drinking fluids and nibbling on snacks on a schedule. (To find out how many carbohydrates you need for recovery, see the sidebar on page 108). And don't forget to drink plenty of water, too! Here are some healthful recovery choices that offer carbohydrate, protein, sodium, and potassium:

- Apple juice + Fig Newtons or oatmeal-raisin cookies + salted almonds or peanuts
- Yogurt + orange juice or fresh fruit + salted pretzels
- Chocolate milk + salted crackers
- Bagel + apple + cheese or peanut butter
- Hot or cold cereal + milk or soymilk + banana or raisins
- Pasta + tomato sauce + meat, seafood, chicken, or cheese
- Pancakes + blueberries + maple syrup
- Fruit + milk + fruit yogurt + a pinch of salt (in a smoothie)
- Vegetable, bean, or noodle soup + bread or crackers + milk
- Small hamburger, soy burger, or turkey sub + orange juice
- Peanut butter and jelly (or honey) sandwich + apple juice
- Baked potato + cheese + ketchup or salsa
- Thick-crust cheese or veggie-cheese pizza

● **RECOVERING FROM A SPECIAL EVENT**—Congratulations! You've completed the event for which you have been training long and hard. Your most important job post-race, post-randonnée, or post-tour is to relax, enjoy yourself, and be proud of your accomplishment. Celebrate with lots of carbohydrates and tasty reward foods.

At this celebratory time, if you have several days before the next event, you need not be obsessive with your recovery diet; you will not be demanding much from your muscles for a while. If you celebrate with beer, wine, or Champagne, be sure to eat first so that you are not drinking alcohol on an empty stomach, and also have some juice or soft drink to supply your muscles with water and carbohydrates. A nice massage and a gentle swim or very light ride to loosen stiff muscles are also good recovery ideas.

● **SUMMARY**—Refueling after hard rides is essential to replenish depleted glycogen and fluid stores, heal damaged muscles, and prepare your body for your next ride.

- Eat or drink carbohydrates within 15 minutes of getting off the bike, and then keep snacking on carbohydrates for the next few hours.
- Drink enough post-ride recovery fluids to quench your thirst, then drink more. Your goal is to have pale-colored urine in significant quantities.
- Eating a little protein with your recovery carbohydrates may enhance glycogen synthesis and muscle repair and reduce muscle soreness, but your focus should remain on carbohydrates and fluid.
- Consume potassium-rich fruits and juices and salty foods and fluids to replace electrolyte losses. While commercial fluid replacement and recovery beverages are convenient, standard foods and fluids can do the job just fine.
- Plan ahead so recovery foods and fluids will be available to you at the end of your ride or workout.
- Enjoy the refueling process...it's part of cycling's pleasures.

As director of the Pan-Mass Challenge, I have noticed that some cyclists, often women, have a hard time eating enough to support their riding. They think food will make them fat. But they need to realize that if they don't eat, they won't perform.

Billy Starr, Boston, MA

CHAPTER 11

Event Week: Nutrition Preparations

I F YOU ARE PREPARING FOR A RACE, TRIATHLON, CENTURY, BREVET, OR any other endurance event that lasts for more than 90 minutes, you should saturate your muscles and liver with glycogen. These stored carbohydrates influence how long you can enjoy exercising. But carbo-loading requires more than just eating a pile of pasta the night before an event. What you do during the week leading up to your important ride can make or break your ability to successfully complete the distance you've been training for.

● **STORED CARBOHYDRATE AND GLYCOGEN**—In comparison to the approximately 1,800 to 2,000 calories stored as carbohydrates, the average, lean 150-pound (70-kilogram) man has 60,000 to 100,000 calories stored as fat, enough to ride several thousand miles! Unfortunately for cyclists and other endurance athletes, fat cannot be used exclusively for fuel because the muscles need carbohydrates to burn fat. Therefore, carbohydrates are a limiting factor for endurance athletes.

The amount of glycogen you use during cycling depends on how hard you ride. Generally speaking, the greater the intensity of the ride, the more glycogen you use. Riding at high intensity, as in all-out sprinting, you burn primarily glycogen; at low intensity, you burn primarily fat. This explains why you may be able to ride casually for several hours, but not

> **"For racing, two days before an event is my most important day. I start drinking more, I make sure to get to bed early, pay close attention to nutrition, and either take the day off or do an easy workout."**
>
> MaryAnn Martinez, Concord, MA

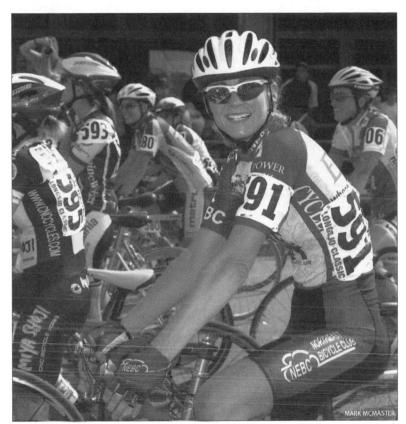

While waiting for your event to start, think positively. Trust that your body is well-fueled, well-trained, and ready to perform at its best.

at a racing pace for more than an hour or two.

When your muscle glycogen stores run out, you will feel exhausted and your physical strength will quickly diminish. When your liver glycogen diminishes, your blood sugar will drop, you will feel irritable, and your mental stamina will rapidly decline. These conditions, known as "hitting the wall" and "bonking," are preventable if you saturate your body with carbohydrates before the ride and also replenish carbohydrates by eating and drinking during the ride. See chapters 8 and 9 for information on fueling before and during rides.

Your muscles' ability to store glycogen increases through training. Well-trained muscles can store 20 percent to 50 percent more glycogen than untrained muscles. This change enhances endurance capacity and is one reason why elite riders can ride for hours without tiring.

• **YOUR DAILY TRAINING DIET**—Pre-event pasta meals have long been a carbo-loading tradition among cyclists. But for optimal glycogen storage, you should carbo-load not just the day before an event but also every day during your training. Cyclists who eat a diet with 55 percent to 65 percent of the calories from carbohydrates can:

- prevent chronic glycogen depletion,
- train better because their muscles are better fueled, and then ride better on event day,
- continue eating the same foods pre-event, so there are no unwanted surprises (the last thing you want to do is change your diet before an event).

Your daily carbo-loading diet should be balanced with an appropriate amount of protein and fat (see chapters 5 and 6). Enjoy grain products, like bread, cereal, pasta, or rice, as the foundation of every meal and snack, along with plenty of fruits and vegetables and smaller amounts of protein foods and dairy products.

To help you avoid nutritional mistakes and reduce unwanted surprises on event day:

- *Practice eating your pre-event meals during training.* If your event will begin in the morning, practice eating breakfast; for afternoon events, breakfast and lunch. If you will be traveling to your race or ride, be sure your tried-and-true foods will be available for event day. You may need to bring all of your foods and drinks with you in a cooler.
- *Train at the time your event will occur.* If your race will start at noon, do some training rides at noon; if your ride will begin at 6:00 a.m., include some early morning rides in your training. Learn how to eat and drink before, during, and after these times.
- *Learn how much pre-exercise food you can eat and then still ride comfortably.* This is particularly important for cyclists who ride at high intensity and have more difficulty digesting and tolerating pre-ride food. These may include racers or those on tour who face a hilly day.
- *Practice drinking the sports drinks and foods that will be available on the ride or at the event as well as any mid-ride foods you plan to eat.* This way, you will know what you can tolerate and what works best for you.

Whether you are at home or at a campsite, the following simple pasta toppings are a change of pace from the standard tomato sauce.

Hot Pasta Ideas

To cooked, hot pasta, add:

- Steamed broccoli or frozen (cooked) mixed vegetables
- Sautéed garlic (in olive oil) + red pepper flakes + chopped tomatoes (sun-dried or fresh)
- Parmesan cheese + chopped herbs (basil, rosemary, oregano) or dry Italian seasonings
- Chicken, shrimp, or scallops sautéed with olive oil, garlic, and a splash of white wine or clam juice
- Canned clams + lemon juice + a little drizzle of olive oil + fresh parsley (or dried herbs)
- Peanut butter heated with a little soy sauce (or hot water to dilute the peanut butter), brown sugar, and ginger
- Chili with kidney beans + cheddar or Jack cheese
- Hummus + cooked broccoli
- Low-fat sour cream + chopped herbs or Italian seasonings + parmesan cheese
- Cooked greens (such as fresh or frozen kale, collards, spinach) + canned white beans + parmesan cheese

Cold Pasta Ideas

To cooked, cooled pasta, add the following. Serve these over lettuce, if desired:

- Low-fat salad dressing of your choice + chopped raw vegetables
- Low-fat Italian dressing mixed with Dijon mustard + tuna + feta cheese + celery + tomatoes
- Garlic and/or fresh ginger, peanut butter, honey, soy sauce (blenderized) + peas or peapods + grated carrot or red bell pepper + tofu (if desired)

Varying the Basic Tomato Sauce

To liven up straight-from-the-jar tomato sauce, try mixing it with:

- A splash or two of red wine
- Cooked turkey sausage, ground beef, or ground turkey
- Cooked chicken tenders
- Sautéed red peppers and onions
- Cooked shrimp or scallops
- A handful of frozen, mixed vegetables, such as broccoli and cauliflower (add directly to heating sauce; cook until heated through)
- Rotisserie or leftover chicken, shredded
- Canned, drained tuna or clams
- Tofu or tempeh cubes or canned beans (drained)
- Fat-free cottage cheese or ricotta cheese + a sprinkle of mozzarella cheese

• THE WEEK BEFORE THE EVENT—The biggest change during the week before an event should be in your training, not in your eating. Taper your training so that your muscles have the opportunity to become fully saturated with glycogen. Do not engage in last-minute hard training that will tap into glycogen stores and burn carbohydrates rather than allow them to be stored. With tapering, the 600 or more calories you would expend during a day's training can be stored as fuel in your muscles and liver. If you are a competitive cyclist who races every weekend or multiple days in a row and have a training schedule that does not allow you to taper, you need to be diligent about maintaining a high-carbohydrate diet and consuming adequate carbohydrates during training and during your events.

Maintain your tried-and-true, high-carbohydrate training diet throughout your taper week. Drastic changes commonly lead to upset stomachs, diarrhea, or constipation. For example, carbo-loading on an unusually high amount of fruits and juices might cause diarrhea; too many white-flour, low-fiber bagels, breads, and pasta might lead to constipation.

Do not worry that you will gain weight and "get fat" during this week of tapering and eating. The extra carbohydrate calories you consume (or rather, that you do not expend) will be stored as glycogen in your liver and muscles. During the weeks and months of athletic training, your muscles have increased their capacity to store glycogen. Your goal with tapering is to fill these large stores to their capacity by eating a carbohydrate-rich, healthful diet. This assures that you will have a full tank of fuel for your event. Now if you are weighing yourself, be forewarned that the scale will go up. This is good! It means you have stored glycogen. For every ounce (28 grams) of carbohydrate stored in your body, you store about three ounces (85 grams) of water. This can translate into three to four pounds (1.5 to 2 kilograms) by the end of your tapering week.

Be sure that you are *carbo*-loading, not *fat*-loading. In the name of carbo-loading, some riders eat dinner rolls slathered

> **❝On race day, I don't eat anything new— my digestive system may not like it. Eating familiar foods makes a real difference in comfort and time spent at checkpoints...or desperately looking for secluded trees! ❞**
>
> John McClellan, Groton, MA

● A CYCLIST'S CARBO-LOADING MENU

Here is an example of a daily carbo-loading menu for a cyclist who weighs 150 pounds (70 kilograms). The menu provides approximately 3,300 calories with 65 percent carbohydrate, adequate protein for muscle repair and maintenance, and limited fat. For more information on the calorie needs of cyclists, refer to chapter 13; for more on protein and fat see chapters 5 and 6, respectively.

Breakfast
1 cup orange juice
1$^1/_2$ cups Cheerios
1 cup low-fat milk
1 medium banana
2 slices whole-wheat toast
1 tablespoon of jelly
2 teaspoons margarine

Lunch
1 medium bagel
1 tablespoon mayonnaise
3 ounces turkey or chicken breast
lettuce and tomato
12 ounces of cranberry-grape juice
6 ounces fat-free blueberry yogurt
6 baby carrots

Snack
12 grapes
$^1/_2$ oz. almonds (roughly 12)

Dinner
2$^1/_2$ cups cooked spaghetti
1 cup tomato sauce
2 ounces cooked, lean ground beef
2 tablespoons grated cheese
$^1/_2$ cup steamed broccoli
1 cup frozen yogurt

Snack
1 cup low-fat milk
6 Fig Newtons

Day's Total:
3,250 calories: 65% carbohydrates, 15% protein, 20% fat

1 cup = 240 milliliters, 1 tablespoon = 15 milliliters; 1 ounce = 28 grams

Nutrition Information from food labels, USDA National Nutrient Database (online), and J. Pennington, 2004, Bowes & Church's Food Values of Portions Commonly Used, 18th ed. (Philadelphia: Lippincott, Williams & Wilkins).

with butter, baked potatoes glistening with butter and sour cream, and rich ice cream. These fatty foods fill the stomach and the fat cells but leave the muscles poorly fueled. This is because dietary fat is not converted to glycogen. If the fat you eat is not needed immediately for energy (for instance, if you will head to the sofa or to bed after eating), it is stored as body fat. The same is true for alcohol. And contrary to popular notion, most of the calories in beer (and wine) come from alcohol, not carbohydrates. Your best bet for carbo-loading is to trade extra fat and alcohol calories for extra carbohydrate calories (see chart on page 122).

Instead of:	Calories	Choose:	Calories
1 roll with butter	200	2 plain rolls or	200
		1 roll with honey or jelly	200
1 cup pasta with oil, cream, or cheese sauce; cheese ravioli, lasagna, or tortellini	250-300	1¹/₂ cups pasta with tomato sauce	250
1 scoop ice cream	200	2 scoops low-fat frozen yogurt	200
Bottle of beer or glass of wine	150	1 cup cranberry juice	150
		or 2 cups fat-free milk	150
		or a can of cola	150
Baked potato with butter/sour cream	300	Baked potato with ketchup or salsa plus extra dinner roll	300

Do not overlook protein-rich foods the days before your event. Endurance athletes burn a little protein for energy and your body requires protein on a daily basis. It is important to eat an appropriate amount of protein every day (see chapter 5). Eat a small serving of low-fat protein such as poached eggs, yogurt, milk, turkey, fish, or chicken as the accompaniment to your meals (do not make protein the main focus), or plant proteins such as beans and lentils (as your intestines can tolerate them).

● **THE DAY BEFORE THE EVENT**—By now, you may have gained about three to four pounds, but don't panic. This weight gain reflects water weight and indicates that your muscles are well-fueled with glycogen. Today is the day to maintain these glycogen stores by enjoying wholesome, carbohydrate-based meals. Don't feel you need to load up with a huge pasta dinner. Instead, why not enjoy a substantial carbo-meal earlier in the day at breakfast or lunch? This allows more time for the food to digest and move through your system. You'll be better off eating a little bit too much than too little on the day before an event. But don't gorge either. Learning the right balance takes practice. Let each preparatory race and long ride be opportunities to learn.

Be sure to drink extra fluids, including water, juices, and soft drinks, to make sure you are fully hydrated. Your urine should be pale yellow and of significant quantity. Abstain from too much wine, beer, and other alcoholic beverages because they can have a dehydrating effect and do not contribute significant carbs.

● **THE MORNING OF THE EVENT**—With luck, you will wake up to a clear, crisp day that makes you want to jump out of bed and jump onto your bike! Before embarking upon your day's task, be sure to eat breakfast. It is the most important meal of the day (see chapter 2). One of the biggest nutritional mistakes made by novice riders and racers is eating too little beforehand, fearing that eating will result in an upset stomach.

As we have mentioned, on your event day be sure to eat only foods and fluids that you have tried and that have worked for you in training. This will help you to avoid unwanted stomach

> **❝If I am doing a century ride the next day, I always fuel up with an early dinner of pasta, chicken, and broccoli the night before. The meal has become a tradition. ❞**
>
> Lenny Sullivan, Methuen, MA

● QUICK AND EASY RICE IDEAS

Here are a few simple and delicious rice suggestions for hungry cyclists.

Cook rice in:
- Chicken, beef, or vegetable broth
- Water or broth + orange or apple juice
- Broth + light coconut milk
- Seasonings· cinnamon, soy sauce, oregano, curry, chili powder, Indian spices, or whatever might nicely blend with the menu

Add cooked rice to:
- Tofu, chicken, or seafood stir-fried with vegetable + soy sauce (or bottle Asian stir-fry sauce)
- Canned or homemade soups and stews
- Bean burritos and tacos
- Vegetable salads

Add to cooked rice:
- Raisins + cashews + curry powder
- Chopped almonds
- Grated fresh lemon peel + black pepper
- Chopped fresh herbs· cilantro, parsley, mint, or basil
- Toasted sesame seeds
- Steamed vegetables + soy sauce
- Mushrooms and peppers, either raw or sautéed
- Low-fat Italian dressing
- Red beans + salsa
- Chili + cheese

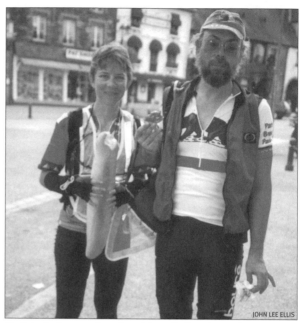

JOHN LEE ELLIS

Cyclists fuel up on bread and jam during the Paris-Brest-Paris brevet. Sticking to familiar, tried-and-true food and beverages that you have tested in training can help assure you energy and success in special events.

and other problems during your ride. If you are used to having a bagel and juice for breakfast, don't feast on pancakes the morning of the ride only to discover that they settle like a lead balloon. You should have learned during training which foods in which amounts your body tolerates before riding. Some cyclists can eat a light breakfast the hour before an event; some even bring food with them to the starting line. Others want six hours for their stomach to empty; they have learned they feel best if they wake up at 4 a.m., eat a bowl of oatmeal, and then go back to bed.

Drink plenty of familiar fluids the morning of the event: water and sports drinks, juices and soft drinks. Water takes 45 to 90 minutes to move through your system, so you can drink several glasses up to two hours before the ride and have time to urinate the excess. Top off your tank with one more glass 5 to 15 minutes before you start riding.

If you are used to having coffee or tea in the morning, do so on event day as well. Some riders drink coffee for mental stimulation or for its laxative effect. Others prefer to abstain because they are already nervous and jittery and have no need for an added buzz. Drinking a mug of hot coffee, warm water with lemon, or hot tea with breakfast stimulates the colon so that you may have a bowel movement, something you might want to achieve before you leave home. Pack extra water, sports drink, latte, juice, soda, or whatever beverages you like (and have tried in training) so they will be available for you at the race or event. Choose what is best for your body, and do what you normally do for your training rides.

- **DURING THE EVENT**—Your job during the ride or race is to prevent dehydration and maintain a normal blood sugar level. Both are essential to maximize your enjoyment and performance during the ride you have been training long and hard for. These topics are discussed in chapters 7, 8, and 9. Remember, do nothing new, special, or different during your event. Stick with what has worked for you and what is familiar to you in your training rides. That is, stick with the tried-and-true, and you will have an enjoyable, well-fueled, and successful ride.

- **SUMMARY**—By event day, you should be well-trained. You should have not only strong muscles but also a strong knowledge of the foods and fluids you need to fuel those muscles. Knowing you are nutritionally prepared, you need not fear that you will tire prematurely. Instead, you can focus on the day's job: completing the distance strongly and successfully with energy to spare!

- As part of your daily training program, you should eat a carbohydrate-rich diet every day. Choose wholesome grain products, such as pasta, rice, whole grain bread, or cereal as the foundation of every meal, along with plenty of fruits and vegetables and smaller amounts of protein and dairy products.

- For competitive endurance events lasting longer than 90 minutes, load your muscles and liver with glycogen days before the event by tapering your training and eating your usual high-carbohydrate sports diet.

- Maintain optimal hydration status by drinking water, juice, soda, or sports drinks. Urine should be pale yellow and of significant quantity.

- To avoid nutrition mistakes and unwanted surprises, try nothing new on event day.

CHAPTER 12

Tips for the Traveling Cyclist

TRAVELING TO ANOTHER CITY, STATE, OR COUNTRY TO PARTICIPATE IN a long ride or race presents its nutritional challenges. The same goes for bike touring. Your food routine is disrupted. You may not have access to foods you are used to eating. And you are confronted with rich temptations that lurk in every restaurant, cafe, and pushcart. All too often you can get sidetracked by the confusion and excitement of being in a new place.

Consuming food or drink that has not been part of your training diet can lead to a number of problems: constipation, stomach upset, diarrhea, gas, dehydration, too few calories,

any of which can hinder your performance and enjoyment on the ride. There is delicious food to be eaten all over the world, and for hungry bikers, it can be tempting to nosh on local fare before or during a ride. If you have an iron stomach, go ahead and enjoy. But for those who want to play it safe and avoid intestinal problems, stick to what you know. You'll ride with confidence knowing that you have eaten your usual sports food, not something new or different that may torment you during the ride!

On a routine day, staying hydrated can be a challenge, but maintaining optimal hydration is even trickier when you are traveling. For one thing, you are not in your usual environment, so water may be inaccessible or you may forget to drink regularly. Plus, riding in a different climate and/or altitude requires you to be even more vigilant about your hydration status. Climate affects your body's cooling system. You may get hotter and require more fluid to stay hydrated. In hot, dry climates, you may sweat more but not realize it because the sweat rapidly evaporates. At higher elevations breathing rate usually increases, resulting in greater water evaporation from your lungs. Stay on top of your hydration by drinking often, taking water with you wherever you go, and drinking on a schedule. (For more on hydration, see chapter 7.)

One key to successfully selecting a top-notch sports diet when you travel is to bring your usual foods and liquids with you. Do not assume the event, venue, hotel, or roadside store will supply you with what you are accustomed to eating. Many organized rides feature food stops along the way that offer anything from familiar peanut butter and jelly to unfamiliar sports bars, gels, and drinks. If you want to try a new sports food or drink, save it for a training ride close to home. This way, you won't risk jeopardizing your comfort and performance by experiencing heartburn, indigestion, or worse.

When traveling, it is easy to become sidetracked by the confusion and excitement of being in a new place. Fight the urge to do too much exploring the day before the ride. Better yet, save the sightseeing and exotic food noshing until after the ride. Allow your muscles to get fully fueled by putting your feet up and resting your legs. Relax with some juices and other tried-and-true carbohydrates, and visualize yourself completing the distance smoothly, strongly, and successfully.

Here are a few tips to help you accommodate a carbohydrate-rich sports diet into your traveling routine.

Breakfast:
- At a restaurant, order pancakes, French toast, whole-wheat toast, bagels, or bran muffins.

> **66** *In my racing days, we saved money when traveling by never eating breakfast out. We'd eat in the hotel room—bagels, fruit, and cereal either brought from home or purchased at a store the night before. My teammate always brought hard-boiled eggs from home. They traveled well in the cooler.* **99**
>
> **Karen Mackin, Acton, MA**

Add honey, jam, or maple syrup for extra carbohydrates. Hold the butter or request that it is served on the side so that you can better control the amount of saturated fat in your meal, or use peanut butter instead.

- Limit cheese omelets, fried potatoes, bacon, biscuits, sausages and other fatty, greasy foods that will leave your muscles unfueled.
- Most restaurants offer cold cereals, oatmeal, and fat-free or low-fat milk, if this is what you prefer in the morning. Add banana, raisins, or brown sugar for more carbohydrates.
- Order a large orange juice or tomato juice. This helps compensate for a potential lack of fruits or vegetables in the other meals.
- For a hotel stay or for early morning events, pack your own cereal, banana or raisins, bowl or cup, spoon, and bottled juice. Bring powdered milk, a milk box (Parmalat or other shelf-stable milk or soymilk), or a cooler with cold milk or yogurt. Or, buy low-fat milk at a local convenience store.

Lunch:

- Find a deli or sandwich shop that offers bagels or wholesome breads. Request a sandwich that emphasizes the bread rather than the filling (preferably lean beef, turkey, ham, or chicken). Limit mayonnaise, butter, or oil-based dressing, and add tomatoes and lettuce. Add more carbohydrates with chocolate low-fat milk, juice, fruit, pretzels, or yogurt (buy these at a convenience store, if the deli doesn't have them).
- At fast-food restaurants, limit the burgers, fried fish, fried chicken, and French fries. They contain a great deal of fat, primarily unhealthful trans or saturated fat. You'll get more carbohydrates by sticking to the spaghetti, baked potatoes, chili, or thick-crust pizza.
- Request thick-crust pizza with vegetable toppings rather than thin-crust pizza with pepperoni or sausage. Blot off the excess grease from the top of the pizza with a few napkins.
- Many supermarkets have salad and soup bars, deli or sandwich counters, and hot meal sections that offer a variety of

healthful and tasty food. While you're there, pick up some yogurt, fruit, juice, bagels, or fig bars for snacks later on.

- At a salad bar, generously pile on the high-carbohydrate items such as chickpeas or other beans, fruit, and starchy vegetables like beets, carrots, and peas. Take plenty of bread. But don't fat-load on butter, salad dressings, and mayonnaise-smothered pasta and potato salads.
- A baked potato is a super choice if you request it plain rather than drenched with butter, sour cream, and cheese toppings. For moistness, mash the potato with some milk (order a glass of milk with your meal), add a tablespoon of sour cream (request it on the side), or top it with ketchup or salsa.
- Choose hearty soups, such as split pea, bean, minestrone, lentil, or noodle, accompanied by crackers, bread, (a plain) bagel, or an English muffin.
- Juices and soft drinks are rich in carbohydrates, but juices are nutritionally preferable for vitamin C, potassium, and wholesome goodness.
- Consider ordering a glass of low-fat or fat-free milk or chocolate milk with your lunch. Often, milk is overlooked as source of carbohydrates, not to mention calcium and protein
- Forgo restaurant food and bring your own lunch fixings. Fill a cooler with: turkey slices or homemade tuna salad, sliced low-fat cheese, peanut butter, baby carrots, cherry tomatoes, apples, low-fat milk, juice, yogurts, and grapes. Pack a loaf of whole-wheat bread or a package of multi-grain bagels, and oatmeal-raisin cookies or dried fruit.

Dinner:

- Check the restaurant beforehand to see if it offers abundant carbohydrates (pasta, baked potatoes, rice, steamed vegetables, salad bar, homemade bread, fruit, and juice) and lower-fat options such as broiled, grilled, or roasted fish, poultry, or meats. Inquire how dishes are made. Request they be prepared with minimal fat.
- Eat the breads and rolls either plain or with jelly or honey. Replace the butter calories with high-carbohydrate choices: another slice of bread, a second potato, soup and crackers, juice, sherbet, or frozen yogurt.

- When ordering salads, always request the dressing be served on the side. Otherwise, you may get as many as 400 calories of oil or mayonnaise, fatty foods that fill your stomach but leave your muscles unfueled.

Snacks:
- Pack your own snacks: pumpernickel bagels, corn muffins, banana bread, rolls, pretzels, fig bars, graham crackers, oatmeal-raisin cookies, granola, oranges, raisins, dried or fresh fruit, and juice boxes.
- Buy wholesome snacks at a convenience or grocery store. Good choices include: trail mix made with nuts and dried fruits, banana, raisins, nuts, cereal bar or granola bar, yogurt, 100% vegetable or fruit juice, bagel or hot pretzel, energy bar, slice of thick-crust pizza, small sandwich, or cup of soup.

- **SUMMARY**–Traveling to cycling events and cycle touring presents nutritional challenges. Not only is your usual food routine disrupted, you are likely to be confronted with rich and tasty temptations that haven't been part of your training diet.
  - Stick to tried-and-true foods and fluids that you know will settle well and not upset your digestive system. That way you'll have no unwanted surprises to ruin your ride.
  - If you have any doubts about the availability of familiar foods, plan ahead and bring some safe foods with you.
  - Pay particular attention to maintaining your hydration by drinking frequently and bringing water with you. It's easy to get sidetracked and forget to drink when you are traveling and having fun.
  - If you want to try a new sports food or drink, try it on a training ride close to home and not on an important ride. This way, you won't risk jeopardizing your comfort and performance. For the same reason, save the exotic food sampling and local foodstuffs for after the ride.

CHAPTER 13

Calculating Your Calorie Needs

Y OU MAY NOT THINK YOU COME CLOSE TO NEEDING THE 6,000 OR more calories that a Tour De France rider needs a day during the famous 21-day stage race. But if you are an active cyclist, you certainly require plenty of calories. Cyclists burn many calories because the sport involves continual hard effort sustained for hours at a time most days of the week. You burn on average 400 to 700 calories an hour on the bike, so you can easily rackup a thousand (or a couple thousand) calories during an afternoon training ride. Long-distance and touring cyclists who ride all day long for days, weeks, or months at a time, can indeed burn as many calories as a racer in the Tour. Physical demands of cycling aside, you are constantly burning calories. You need calories simply to exist: to breathe, blink, pump blood, and yes, to click the television remote control on recovery days.

> ❝ **The worst nutritional mistake I have made was assuming biking allowed me to eat whatever I wanted, and not gain weight.** ❞
>
> Rich Lesnik, San Francisco, CA

● **COUNTING CALORIES**—Most cyclists can naturally regulate a proper calorie intake and have little need to count calories. They eat when they are hungry and stop when they are content. Others have lost touch with their body's ability to regulate an appropriate food intake—they may deny themselves food when they are hungry (as often happens with reducing diets), but then overeat later on.

Counting calories can help erratic eaters and dieters to get

By using the following formula, you can estimate your personal calorie needs and gain a perspective on how to balance calories eaten versus calories expended.*

1. To estimate your resting metabolic rate, that is, the amount of calories you need to simply breathe, pump blood, and be alive, multiply your weight by 10 calories per pound (or 22 calories per kilogram). (If you are significantly over-weight, use a weight that is halfway between your desired weight and your current weight.) So, if you weigh 150 pounds (70 kilograms), you need approximately 1,500 calories simply to do nothing all day except exist:

   150 pounds x 10 calories/pound = 1,500 calories

2. Add more calories for activities of daily living *apart from your riding* and other purposeful exercise (see note below). Add:
   - 30 to 40 percent if you are mostly sedentary (sitting, typing, reading, resting, or taking it easy to recover from a ride);
   - 50 percent if you are moderately active (frequently standing and walking, doing household chores, moving often throughout the day); or
   - 60 to 70 percent or more if you are mostly or very active (sitting very little, working/walking on your feet most of the day).

If you weigh 150 pounds (70 kilograms) and are moderately active when you are not riding, you would add 50 percent to your resting metabolic rate (1,500 calories), or 750 calories, for activities of daily living. So, you may need 2,200 calories in a day total without riding:

1,500 calories + 50% (or 750 calories) = 2,250 (let's say 2,200) calories a day

Note: For long-distance riders, the number of calories used for activities of daily living may actually be very small (because they are riding for most of the day and because they tend to be sedentary once they're off the bike). So when calculating your calorie needs for long-ride days, use a lower activity level so that you do not overestimate the total number of calories you burn in a day.

3. Now, add more calories for your riding and other purposeful exercise. Refer to the chart on page 138. If you weigh 150 pounds (70 kilograms) and you ride consistently hard at 15 miles per hour without drafting for 1.5 hours, you burn approximately 1000 calories while riding. This brings your day's total calorie needs to approximately 3,200 calories:
   - 150 pounds x 4.5 calories/pound/hour (see chart, page 138) = 675 calories/hour
   - 675 calories/hour x 1.5 hour = 1,013 calories for the ride (let's say 1,000)
   - 1,000 calories + 2,200 calories = 3,200 total calories/day with 1.5 hours of riding

4. If you want to lose weight, subtract approximately 20 percent of your total calorie needs. If you want to gain, add 20 percent. If your daily calorie needs are 3,200 on ride days and you want to lose weight, subtract 600 calories or so from 3,200. This gives you a total of 2,600 calories a day to lose weight (on rest days subtract 440 calories from 2,200 for about 1,800 calories a day):

3,200 calories – 20% (or roughly 600 calories) = 2,600 calories per day for weight loss on ride days

5. Finally, divide your day's calorie budget evenly into three or four parts of the day: morning, noon/afternoon, and evening. For example:

Meal	Calories Ride days	Calories Rest days
Breakfast/snack	1,000	700
Lunch/snack	1,000	800
Dinner/snack	1,000	700
During 1.5 hour ride	200	
Total	3,200	2,200

Note. On ride days you may not feel hungry enough to eat this much, and on rest days you may be ravenous and want to eat more. Remember to listen to your appetite: eat when hungry and stop when content. To lose weight, stop eating when you are almost content

6. Read food labels to become familiar with the calorie content of the foods you commonly eat and then balance your calorie budget according to the rules for a well-balanced diet.

Here are approximate calorie needs for cyclists of different weights who are moderately active throughout the day**:

Weight lbs (kg)	daily living	Approximate calorie needs for: (ride speeds are not with drafting) + 2-hour ride at 11 mph (18 km/hr)	+ 2-hour ride at 15 mph (24 km/hr)	+ 2-hour ride at 18 mph (29 km/hr)
120 (55)	1,800	+600 = 2,400	+ 1,100 = 2,900	+1,300 = 3,100
140 (64)	2,100	+700 = 2,800	+ 1,300 = 3,400	+1,550 = 3,650
160 (73)	2,400	+800 = 3,200	+ 1,450 = 3,850	+1,750 = 4,150
180 (82)	2,700	+900 = 3,600	+ 1,650 = 4,350	+1,950 = 4,650

*These guidelines do not address the needs of each individual. For personalized calorie information you should meet with a registered dietitian who specializes in sports nutrition. Contact the American Dietetic Association at (800) 366-1655 to find a sports nutritionist in your area, or visit their website at www.eatright.org and use the convenient referral network.

**Calorie expenditure information from Ainsworth et al., 2000.

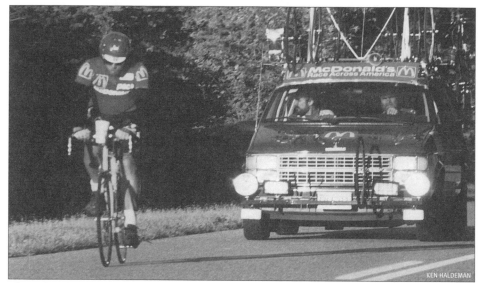

Ultracycling champion Lon Haldeman targets nearly 12,000 calories a day during the grueling 3,000-mile Race Across America (RAAM). Knowing how many calories your body needs and eating on a schedule can help you to fuel appropriately during long rides, particularly if you do not feel hungry while riding.

in touch with appropriate portion sizes and acknowledge how they feel when they are appropriately fed. Once educated about how much is appropriate to eat, they can then learn how to better regulate their food intake without counting calories. Calorie information can also help touring cyclists, randonneurs, and other long-distance cyclists who may not feel hungry while riding to fuel themselves adequately on long rides.

> **❝I figure I double my calorie intake when I'm touring...No hardship there! ❞**
>
> Candace Crowell, Georgetown, MA

● **HONOR HUNGER**—Generally, the more you exercise, the hungrier you will get. Whereas most cyclists honor their hunger by refueling with wholesome meals, others feel confused by hunger and sometimes even feel guilty that they are always eager to eat. Hunger is not bad or wrong. It is simply your body's way of telling you it needs more fuel; you should respond appropriately by eating.

You should not spend your day feeling hungry, weak, and tired, even if you are trying to lose weight (see chapter 14). If your 8 a.m. breakfast finds you hungry earlier than 11 a.m., your breakfast simply contained too few calories. You need to

THE CYCLIST'S FOOD GUIDE: FUELING FOR THE DISTANCE

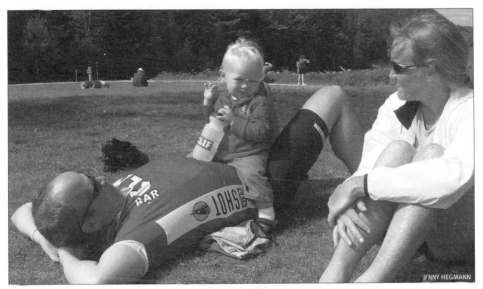

Toddlers have the natural ability to eat when they are hungry and stop when they are content. Many adults have lost this ability, but can relearn how to eat appropriately.

eat either a bigger breakfast or a midmorning snack. If you are hungry all afternoon, starving by dinnertime, and overeating in the evening, you clearly are not eating enough during the day.

Cyclists need good food on a regular schedule. Think of your day's calorie needs in terms of an accounting system and add in calories as you burn them. You should plan to eat at least every four hours during the day and allot about one-fourth of your day's calories for each section of the day (morning, midday, afternoon and evening). This balance sheet approach can be particularly helpful to cyclists who feel tired or hungry all the time or lack energy for workouts or for those who are trying to change their weight.

> ❝I eat often, every two to three hours, to keep my energy level up. Three meals alone would never do! ❞
> MaryAnn Martinez, Concord, MA

If you prefer to satisfy your appetite with three big meals or multiple mini-meals in a day, that's fine. Just eat evenly, on a schedule. For example, if you like to eat a light breakfast, then eat a second breakfast midmorning to satisfy your energy needs. Come midday, enjoy lunch as being the second-most-important meal of the day. (Morning riders need a hearty lunch to refuel their muscles; afternoon riders need a respectable lunch for their

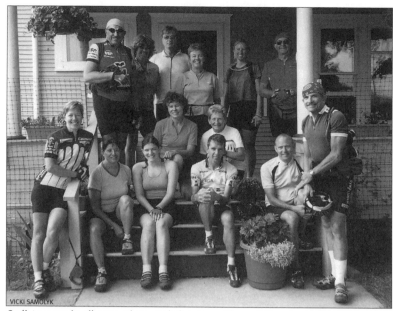

Cyclists come in all ages, sizes, and shapes and have different calorie requirements. But by honoring hunger, each cyclist can fuel optimally for high energy.

after-work ride.) Enjoy a second lunch later in the afternoon (to fuel-up for your after-work training) and then a wholesome dinner in the evening (to refuel from your busy day). If you won't be home for your usual dinnertime, then plan to eat a substantial part of your dinner calories in the afternoon.

If this sounds like a lot of daytime food to you, you may be eating backwards. That is, if you do most of your eating in the evening and battle hunger all day, stop! Move some of those evening calories to the daytime, so you will have more energy during the day when you need it most. Your workouts will be stronger, you will feel more energetic and awake, and you won't be distracted by constant hunger.

● **CALORIES FOR CYCLING—**The following chart gives an approximation of the calories used during activities bicyclists often enjoy. Keep in mind that the precise number of calories burned by an individual can be measured only with

> **❝I've finally learned to eat enough food during the day. I feel so much stronger all the time. I've actually lost weight while eating more food—but the secret is to eat more good food, not junk food. ❞**
>
> Tracie Timothy, Salt Lake City, UT

special metabolic equipment in a well-controlled lab setting. Calorie expenditure depends on many factors, including your fitness level, age, gender, and, of course, how hard you ride. You burn many more calories when you ride uphill, with a heavy load, or into the wind than when you ride downhill, unencumbered, or with a tailwind. Racers know that they can conserve energy by drafting behind other riders in the pack. Also, body position affects how many calories you burn: Standing on the pedals burns more calories than sitting with hands on brake hoods, which burns more calories than sitting, tucked in the aero position.

On ride days, you burn many more calories than on days you do not ride. If you weigh 150 pounds (70 kilograms) you need approximately 2,200 calories on non-ride days and 3,600 calories on ride days (two hours of moderately hard riding means approximately 1,400 additional calories). This can present a dilemma: How do you eat an additional 1,400 calories in a day?

If you are eating appropriately, the 200 or so calories you consume before and during each hour of riding and your recovery meal will help you meet your calorie needs on ride days. In addition, riding makes you hungry (sooner or later, if not during or immediately afterward), so you will naturally want to eat more on that day or the next day. Calorie intake fluctuates day-to-day whether we are aware of it or not. On ride days you might eat fewer calories than you burn, but on the next day you may end up feeling hungrier and eating more than usual. This extra food will be used to recover your body and replenish depleted glycogen stores. You should honor your hunger and regularly eat nutritious food. If your weight is not changing and you feel energetic overall, you are meeting your calorie requirements. Eating for riding is discussed more thoroughly in chapters 8, 9, and 10.

Wise caloric spending is the key to performance and good health. Remember to choose a variety of healthful, wholesome

> **"Two days after I finished my TransAmerica tour, I became a graduate student. My activity dropped from six (or more) hours of daily cycling to sedentary. I had fears I would get fat because I'd want to keep eating like a touring cyclist. But my hearty appetite disappeared and I was content to eat less, without feeling denied or deprived."**
>
> Nancy Clark, West Newton, MA

To estimate how many calories you use during an activity:

Take your weight and multiply it by the calories used per hour of activity. Then multiply that number by how many hours (or fractions of hours) during which you maintained the activity. For example, a 150-pound (70-kilogram) cyclist who rides at an average pace of 15 miles per hour (24 kilometers per hour) for 1.5 hour alone (not drafting) will burn approximately 1000 calories during that activity:

150 lb x 4.5 cal/lb/hr = 675 cal/hr; 675 cal/hr x 1.5 hr = 1013 calories

Bicycling: *Calories used per pound or kilogram of body weight per hour*

Speed	Description	cal/lb/hr	cal/kg/hr
11 mph (18 km/hr)	leisure, slow, light effort	2.5	6
13 mph (21 km/hr)	leisure, moderate effort	3.5	8
15 mph (24 km/hr)	racing or leisure, fast, vigorous effort	4.5	10
16-19 mph (26-31 km/hr)	racing, not drafting, fast	5.5	12
›19 mph (31 km/hr)	racing, drafting, very fast	5.5	12
› 20 mph (32 km/hr)	racing, not drafting, very fast	7.5	16
unspecified	mountain, cross, or BMX biking	4	8.5

Other Activities: *Calories used per pound or kilogram of body weight per hour*

Description	cal/lb/hr	cal/kg/hr
Hockey, field or ice	3.5	8
Lying awake or sitting quietly, watching TV, reading	0.5	1
Running, 6 mph (10 km/hr)	4.5	10
Running, 10 mph (16 km/hr)	7.5	16
Skiing, cross-country, 2.5 mph (4 km/hr), light effort	3	7
Skiing, cross-country, 5-8 mph (8-13 km/hr), vigorous effort	4	9
Skiing, cross-country, ›8 mph (13 km/hr), racing, hard effort	6.5	14
Skiing, downhill, light effort	2	5
Skiing, downhill, vigorous effort, racing	3.5	8
Sleeping	0.4	0.9
Soccer, casual, general	3	7
Stretching, Hatha yoga	1	2.5
Swimming, freestyle, fast, vigorous effort	4.5	10
Swimming, freestyle, slow, moderate effort	3	7
Walking, level surface, 3 to 4 mph (4.5 to 6.5 km/hr)	1.5-2.5	3.5-5
Weight lifting (free, Nautilus- or Universal-type), body building, vigorous effort	2.5	6

Adapted from Ainsworth BE, et al, 2000.

foods for meals, snacks, and exercise-related fuel. And if occasionally you want to splurge on a decadent dessert or post-ride ice-cream sundae, that's okay as long as your overall diet is sensible. Refer to chapter 1 for information on how to balance your diet.

• SUMMARY—

- Hungry cyclists need good, wholesome food on a regular schedule so they can enjoy an even flow of energy throughout the day. You should plan to eat every four hours or more often.
- Knowing how many calories you need can help you to eat enough to fuel your cycling, avoid being hungry all day long, plan your meals appropriately, and achieve your weight goals.
- Hunger is not bad or wrong; it's simply your body's request for fuel. Honor hunger by eating nourishing foods when your body requests fuel.
- Fueling before, during, and after riding will help you to meet the caloric demands of cycling. Feeling hungrier on the days you ride, or the day after, is normal and allows you to eat enough to support your training and refueling program.

"Usually, I just eat when I am hungry...and I notice being extra hungry after an intense race, or extra long (century) ride. In that case, I just eat more!"

Karen Mackin, Acton, MA

CHAPTER 14

How to Lose Weight and Have Energy to Ride

EXERCISE BURNS CALORIES, AND THAT IS ONE OF THE REASONS WHY people bike, run, and enjoy other forms of physical activity. Consistent exercise helps them manage their weight and allows more freedom with eating. But for many active people weight remains a significant issue. There are plenty of cyclists who are in a constant battle with their weight and feel frustrated that they just can't seem to shed those final few pounds. Inevitably, the first words they say are, "I know what to do to lose weight. I just can't do it." They think they should follow a strict diet with rigid rules and regulations. Wrong. Diets don't work. If diets did work, everyone would be as thin as desired. The key to losing weight is to stop thinking about going on a diet and start learning how to eat healthfully.

● **HOW MUCH IS OKAY TO EAT?**—To determine just how much you can appropriately eat, refer to the previous chapter. Note that your body requires a large amount of energy to simply exist—to pump blood, breathe, produce urine, and grow hair. Also note that you deserve to eat those maintenance calories even if you are injured and unable to ride.

An appropriate reducing diet knocks off only

> 66 **Over the winter off-season, my body fat increases somewhat. Come springtime, I work to lose that extra body fat by cutting out refined carbs and sweets, like muffins and cookies, and eating more fruits, whole grains, and vegetables. That, combined with increased time on the bike, works for me.** 99
>
> MaryAnn Martinez, Concord, MA

20 percent of your calorie needs. To do this, you need to know not only how many calories your body requires but also how many calories you're eating. Let's take a look at Jane, a 120-pound (55-kilogram) graduate student, who exercised for an hour on most days. She required about 2,200 to 2,300 calories to maintain her weight:

- 1,200 calories for her resting metabolic rate (10 calories per pound x 120 pounds) +
- 600 calories for general activity (50% x 1,200 calories) +
- 500 calories for an hour of cycling (4.0 calories/pound/hour x 120 pounds).

To appropriately lose weight, she needed to cut her total calorie intake by 20 percent (about 400 to 500 calories), leaving her with 1,800 calories for her diet plan.

To Jane, 1,800 sounded like too many calories. She exclaimed "I could never eat that much; I'd gain weight! If I can't lose weight eating only 1,000 calories a day, how could I possibly lose

❝ It's always a battle to not overeat when you're a pro cyclist—to stop when you're full and not go on eating because it tastes good, or you don't want to waste any food, or you're bored. If I stop when I'm full, I'm usually proud of myself, sated, and in a good mood. ❞

Adam Hodges Myerson,
Northampton, MA

weight eating 1,800 calories? My metabolism is so slow…"

Although Jane challenged the calorie recommendations, Nancy suggested that she keep an open mind. The latest research on athletes' calorie needs suggests that very few athletes actually do have slow metabolisms. Researchers have even studied active people like Jane who claim to maintain weight despite eating next to nothing. When carefully monitored, these women burned the calories one would expect based on standard calculations. Their metabolisms were fine, but they had problems acknowledging how much food they actually ate. Their nibbles on bagels, apples, rice cakes, and broken cookies added up! For more information, refer to *Slow Metabolism Woes* in chapter 16.

Because Jane claimed she ate far less than her peers, she needed to heighten her awareness of her food intake by keeping food records to track everything she ate. Food records can be extremely useful to help you understand your eating habits. You might notice that you:

- Eat when reading and don't even notice the portion
- Eat too little at breakfast and lunch, only to overeat at night
- Diet Monday through Thursday, then splurge on weekends

Research indicates that keeping accurate food records can help people lose weight. By knowing what and when you eat, why you eat, and where you eat, you can take the necessary steps to eat 20 percent less, an appropriate reducing diet.

• FIVE KEYS TO SUCCESSFUL WEIGHT REDUCTION—If you want to lose weight healthfully and keep it off, we suggest you calculate your calorie needs (see the previous chapter) and follow these five recommendations.

Key #1. Eat enough. Don't get too hungry or you will blow your diet. Many weight-conscious cyclists try to eat as little as possible. That's a big mistake. Perhaps the following case study will help you understand why. Cindi thought skimping on food was a good way to diet and she felt frustrated by her lack of weight loss. She explained, "I have only coffee for breakfast. I exercise at lunchtime and then just eat a salad with cottage cheese. Nighttime is my trouble-time. I just cannot seem to stay away from the frozen yogurt...It seems the more I diet, the more weight I gain."

Clearly, not eating was Cindi's problem. Dieting and denial were getting her nowhere. She needed to accept that she is supposed to eat and to trust that appropriate eating will contribute to an appropriate weight.

In trying to stick to her bare-bones diet, Cindi's breakfast and lunch totaled less than a quarter of the 2,400 calories she required. It is no wonder that she lacked energy for her workouts and was starving by dinnertime! She would often skip her training sessions and then at night eat everything in sight, only to get up the next morning with a food hangover. She would then vow to get back on her diet, skip breakfast, skimp on lunch, lack energy to enjoy exercise, and blow her diet again at night. Although Cindi deserved a lot of credit for having the willpower to survive the day on so few calories, her method was mistaken. Her diet was too strict.

If you, like Cindi, are trying to lose weight by eating as little as possible and exercising as hard as you can, remember that the less you eat, the more likely you are to blow your diet. Even if you can successfully restrict your intake, the less you eat, the more your body adjusts to having fewer calories. You will start to hibernate similar to what a bear does in winter when food is scarce. Your metabolic rate will drop to conserve calories and you will feel lethargic, cold, and lack energy to pedal strongly through a workout.

Research comparing sedentary dieters who either crash-dieted on 500 calories per day or followed a more reasonable reducing

> **For a while I was trying to eat less so that I could weigh less, but I'd end up eating more and weighing more. I finally learned that if I eat sensibly—three meals per day—that my weight is fine. I feel better and exercise better.**
> Candace Strobach, Kinnelon, NJ

> **I have no doubt that when I diet and try to lose weight too fast, my performance suffers.**
> Ryan Fletcher, Denver, CO

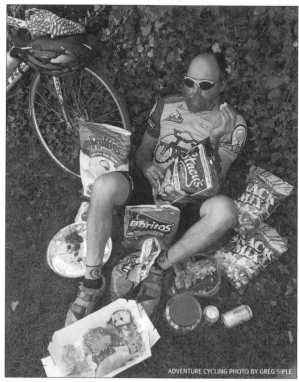
ADVENTURE CYCLING PHOTO BY GREG SIPLE

Eating enough during the daytime and during rides helps you to avoid the extreme hunger that can lead to food cravings, overeating less-than-stellar food choices, and undesired weight gain.

plan of 1,200 calories showed that both groups lost a similar amount of body fat. The crash diet, however, caused the metabolic rate to drop by 17 percent (Foster et al. 1990). Why bother to eat next to nothing when you can lose weight with eating just 20 percent less than you need to maintain your weight?

Most female cyclists who want to lose weight should follow 1,800- to 2,200-calorie (or greater) reduction diets, depending on how hard they train. This is far more than most 800- to 1,200-calorie diets that are designed for sedentary people who can get away with eating very little. You need a substantial amount of energy to fuel your muscles and have energy to enjoy your training.

Key #2. Be sure that you eat more during the day, so that you will be able to eat less (diet) at night. For an appropriate reducing program, divide your calories evenly throughout the day. Keep in mind that athletes tend to get hungry (and should eat) at least every four hours. A 150-pound (70-kilogram) cyclist who is on a 2,200-calorie reducing diet may plan the day as such:

Breakfast:	8 a.m.	600 calories
Lunch:	Noon	600 calories
Snack:	4 p.m.	400 calories
Ride 1 hour:	6 p.m.	
Dinner:	8 p.m.	600 calories

Your goal is to eat on a schedule to prevent yourself from getting too hungry.

Your training program may require creative meal scheduling if you exercise during meal times. For example, if you ride at 6 p.m., potentially at the height of your hunger, you might better enjoy your training if you eat part of your dinner beforehand. You could trade in your 200-caloric dinner potato for a 200 calorie bagel at 4 p.m. Similarly, if you ride at 6 a.m., you might enjoy greater energy if you eat part of your breakfast beforehand, such as a slice of toast and a glass of juice, and then eat the rest afterwards to recover and to satisfy your hunger. As mentioned in chapter 8, you need to experiment with pre-exercise food to determine the right amount of calories to boost your energy without making you feel heavy and sluggish.

Some cyclists believe that riding "on empty," such as riding first thing in the morning without having eaten, burns more body fat than exercising well-fueled. While this is true, keep in mind that *burning* body fat does not equate to *losing* body fat. To have a net loss of body fat, you need to create and maintain a calorie deficit; you need to burn more calories than you consume over a period of days. People who exercise on empty usually do not achieve net fat loss because they have difficulty creating and maintaining a calorie deficit:

- They lack the energy for long, strong workouts, and end up burning fewer calories than someone who is properly fueled before exercise.

> **"To lose weight I used to hold back on eating, then go out and push myself on the bike. Afterward, I'd reward myself with a huge meal. Now, I eat before and during the ride to fuel the ride, and I don't deal with hunger afterwards. I have lost weight and I ride stronger."**
>
> Rich Lesnik, San Francisco, CA

• They experience extreme hunger later on, which can lead to overeating calories.

Key #3. Eat an appropriate amount of fat. If you currently eat a high-fat diet filled with butter, mayonnaise, salad dressing, greasy meals, and rich desserts, you should cut back on these fattening foods. Excess dietary fat easily turns into excess body fat, if not clogged arteries.

But some of today's bikers try to totally avoid fat. They think that if they eat fat, they will instantly get fat. This is not always the case. Some fat in your food may actually help you lose weight. Take a look around and notice the number of trim cyclists whose diets include some fat. If you are trying to knock all the fat out of your diet, think again.

• commonly feel hungry, denied, deprived,

• feel guilty when they inevitably "cheat" by eating fat, and

• eat an unbalanced diet that may be too low in protein and can hurt their performance.

One study showed that dieters who were taught to eat 1,200 calories of a standard American (35-percent-fat) diet actually lost more body fat than the group who were taught to eat 1,200 calories of a low-fat (20-percent-fat) diet (McManus et al. 2001). Why? Because the high-fat dieters were better able to comply with their regimen. Fat is helpful for dieters because it takes longer to digest and provides a nice feeling of satisfaction that can prevent you from searching through the kitchen for something tasty to eat. Fat is also needed to absorb certain vitamins.

You will enjoy more success with losing body fat if you give yourself a reasonable calorie and fat budget to spend on the foods that you want to eat. By choosing the 25-percent-fat diet that is described in chapter 6, you can add a little fat to each meal, provide your body with important nutrients, feel more satisfied, and be better able to stick to your diet. For generations, people have lost fat even though their diets included fat. You can too!

Key #4. You don't have to lose weight every day. Losing weight requires enough mental energy to tell yourself, "I'd rather be thinner than eat more calories." Some days you may lack that mental energy. For example, Jim, a stockbroker who wanted to lose five pounds before an Ironman triathlon, was stressed out by his demanding workload, training schedule, and family problems. Although he wanted to drop a few pounds, he lacked the mental energy he needed to cut calories. At the end of the day, he'd inevitably succumb to cookies. It seemed like a nice reward for having survived the day, but it also contributed to weight gain. Jim needed to be reminded that he is only human, with a limited amount of mental and physical energy. Rather than punish himself for lacking energy to diet, he needed to accept the fact that he was stressed and in need of comfort. Like it or not, food provided that comfort

Jim needed to let go of his current goal to lose fat and focus instead on maintaining his weight and fueling his muscles appropriately. Well-fueled muscles would enhance his training more

---

● WHY ARE YOU EATING?

Food has many roles. It satisfies hunger, fuels muscles, is a pleasurable part of social gatherings and celebrations, rewards us at the end of a stressful day, and has a calming effect. If you tend to eat for reasons other than fuel, think HALT and ask yourself: Why do I want to eat? Is it because I am...
- Hungry?
- Angry or Anxious?
- Lonely?
- Tired?

If you are eating inappropriately, remember that no amount of food will solve any problem. Don't start eating if you know you will have problems stopping.

than would poorly fueled muscles, especially if they were depleted from improper dieting. Jim was in a stressful season in his life, and he needed to remove the additional self-imposed stress of trying to lose weight. He reluctantly agreed with that reality.

Stressful times are often poor times to try to reduce body fat. Instead, you should focus on exercising regularly to help cope with stress and on eating healthfully to prevent the weight gain that sometimes occurs during stressful times. Note that cyclists who are both stressed and hungry can easily succumb to overeating, so it can be helpful to eat every four hours to keep your appetite at bay. Of course, no amount of food will solve any problem; it only adds to your feeling out of control.

Key #5. Have realistic weight goals. Weight is more than just a matter of willpower. Genetics plays a large role. If you are eating appropriately during the day, exercising regularly, eating lighter at night, and waking up eager for breakfast but still have not lost weight, perhaps you have an unrealistic goal. It is possible that you have no excess fat to lose and you are already very lean for your genetic blueprint. Every body is different, but any body can be fit. Just take a look around at a bike race, tour, or ride and you will see all body types, from slight and sinewy to broad and muscle-bound. Like it or not, nature may want you to look more like a linebacker, than the narrow, lightweight Lance Armstrong you may wish to be.

> **"Do not be obsessed with the numbers on the scale. With time and training, you will learn at what weight you can perform well. Listening to your body is more accurate than any scale."**
>
> Mike Czech, Edison, NJ

Women cyclists in particular complain about their natural physiques, that biking makes their legs and butts bigger. Many wish their tight-fitting riding shorts better disguised their round hips and jiggly upper thighs. Earlier in this chapter, we mentioned Cindi, who was skimping on food, trying to eat as little as possible in her struggle to lose weight. Cindi was short and had thin hair and big thighs, just like her mothers and sisters. Although she put no effort into trying to grow taller or thicken her hair, she obsessed about the fat on her thighs and spent lots of energy trying to reduce them.

THE CYCLIST'S FOOD GUIDE: FUELING FOR THE DISTANCE

Cindi needed to know that although she could remodel her body to a certain extent, she could not totally redesign it. Plain and simple, active people and athletes come in varying sizes and shapes. No single body type is right or wrong.

In order to determine an appropriate weight for your body, stop looking at the scale and start looking at your family. Imagine yourself at a family reunion:

- How do you compare to other members of your family?
- Are you currently leaner than they are? fatter? the same?
- If leaner, are you straining to stay that way?
- If you are significantly leaner, you may already be underfat for your body.

Many people, cyclists and non-athletes alike, put their lives on hold, struggling to lose a final few pounds. As Cindi said as she grabbed onto her thighs, "I hate being seen in my shorts. But no matter how much I exercise, I can't get rid of these fat thighs. I must be doing something wrong." Cindi was simply trying to get to a weight that was abnormal for her genetics. She was already leaner that other members of her family.

She needed to understand the reason why women as compared to men have fat thighs: The fat in the hips, buttocks, and thighs is sex-specific. It is a storehouse of energy for potential pregnancy and breast-feeding and is supposed to be there. Just as women have breast tissue, women also have hip, buttock, and thigh tissue. Women have fatter derrieres and legs than men because women are women. Bicycling works the leg, gluteal, and hip muscles, so bikers should expect to gain muscle mass in those areas. But that doesn't change the fact that nature wants women to have some fat in those areas too. The result can be, yes, bigger thighs and butts, but also stronger muscular pistons to power you mile after mile. Cindi needed to accept the realities of being a woman and stop comparing herself to the magazine and catalog models who do indeed have rare physiques. For more on women's issues, see chapter 16.

If you are wasting time complaining about your body, keep in perspective:

- Life is a gift.
- Life is too short to be spent obsessing about food and weight.

    Yes, you do want to be fit and healthy, but you need not

strive to be sleek and skinny. The cost attached to achieving the perfect weight and the perfect body is often yo-yo dieting, poor nutrition, lack of energy to ride well, guilt for eating, a sense of failure that can play havoc with your self-esteem, and poor cycling performance. Love your body for what it is. Stop hating it for what it is not.

● **SUMMARY**—Food is fuel, healthful, and health-giving. You are supposed to eat even if you are trying to lose weight. Be realistic about your weight-loss expectations and remember:

- The thinnest rider may not be the fastest rider.
- The best-fueled rider will always win with good nutrition.
- You are supposed to eat even if you want to lose body fat. Deduct only 20 percent of your calorie budget, but do not starve yourself.
- You should eat during the day, and then diet at night. Early morning hunger is a sign you did not overeat the night before.
- Your diet should include a little bit of fat to keep you feeling satisfied, to help provide you with important nutrients, and fuel long rides.
- Realize that you do not have to lose weight every day; stress-filled days can be for maintaining weight.
- Be realistic with your weight goals. You may have no weight to lose, according to your genetics.

CHAPTER 15

How to Gain Weight Healthfully

IF YOU ARE AMONG THE MINORITY OF CYCLISTS WHO STRUGGLE WITH being too thin, food may seem a medicine, meals a burden, and the expense of food budget-breaking. Through discipline and diet, you can change your physique to a certain extent, but first, you must have a clear picture of your genetic blueprint and a realistic goal:

- What do other people in your family look like?
- Was your mother or father very slim at your age?
- When did she or he gain weight?
- What does she or he look like now?

If at your age a parent was equally thin, you probably are genetically predisposed to be thin and may have trouble adding pounds. For example, in a classic study on identical twins, some pairs of twins gained more weight than others, even though everyone overate by an equal amount, 1,000 extra calories per day (Bouchard 1991). Researchers aren't sure why some people are "hard gainers." The body may adjust its metabolism to maintain a predetermined genetic weight, and people who fidget more may burn significantly more calories (Levine et al. 2000).

● **SIX RULES FOR GAINING WEIGHT**—To gain weight, the bottom line is you have to consume more calories than you expend. There is no instant cure or magic solution. If you are a hard gainer, you may require a significant amount of calories to add weight. Adding muscle-building exercise, such as weightlifting, helps convert the extra calories into muscle rather than fat.

Underweight cyclists should consume an additional 500 to 1,000 calories per day. If you are committed to the weight-gain process, you can expect to gain one-half to one pound per week.

The trick to successful weight gain is to pay careful attention to these six important rules.

1. Eat consistently. Have three hearty meals plus one or two additional snacks daily. Do not skip meals. You may not feel hungry for lunch if you have eaten a big breakfast, but you should eat regardless. Otherwise, you will miss out on important calories you need to accomplish your goal.

2. Eat larger portions. Some people think they need to buy expensive weight-gain powders. Not true. Standard food works fine. The only reason commercial powders "work" is because they provide additional calories. If you drink the recommended three glasses per day of a 300-calorie weight-gain shake, you will consume an extra 900 calories and likely achieve the desired results. But you could less expensively consume those extra calories by eating more of readily available foods, such as:
- A bigger bowl of cereal
- A larger piece of fruit
- An extra sandwich for lunch or a large sub sandwich
- Two potatoes or two rolls at dinner instead of one
- A taller glass of milk or juice

3. Select higher-calorie foods, but not higher-fat foods. Excess fat calories easily convert into body fat that fattens you up rather than bulks up your muscles. The best bet for extra calories is to choose carbohydrate-rich foods that have more calories than an equally enjoyable counterpart. For instance, an eight-ounce (240-milliliter) glass of cranberry juice has 170 calories whereas the same amount of grapefruit juice has only 100 calories. Extra carbohydrates will give you the energy you need to do muscle-building exercise. By reading food labels, you can make the best choices. See *How to Boost Your Calories* on the next page.

4. Drink extra juice and low-fat milk. Beverages are a simple way to increase caloric intake. Instead of drinking primarily

● HOW TO BOOST YOUR CALORIES

To consume more calories, choose foods and beverages that contain more calories per serving, such as those suggested here. Calorie information is for a one-cup (240-milliliter) serving, unless otherwise noted.

Choose more:	Calories	Instead of:	Calories
Cranberry juice	170	Orange juice	110
Grape juice	160	Grapefruit juice	100
Banana, 1 large	170	Apple, 1 large	130
Granola	380	Bran flakes	120
Grape-Nuts	410	Cheerios	90
Corn	140	Green beans	40
Carrots	45	Zucchini	30
Split pea soup	130	Vegetable soup	80
Baked beans	260	Rice	190
Chocolate low-fat (1%) milk	160	Low-fat (1%) milk	100

water, quench your thirst with caloric containing fluids. One high school athelete, a client of Nancy's, gained 13 pounds over the summer by simply adding six glasses of cranberry-apple juice (about 1,000 calories) to his standard daily diet. Extra juices are not only a great source of calories and fluids but also carbohydrates to keep muscles well-fueled and ready to ride.

5. *Do strength training.* Also called resistance training or weightlifting, this type of exercise stimulates muscular develop-ment, so that you bulk up instead of fatten up. Note that extra exercise, not extra protein, is the key to muscular development. If you are concerned the extra exercise will result in weight loss rather than weight gain, remember that exercise tends to stimu-late the appetite. Yes, a hard ride or training session may tem-porarily "kill" your appetite right after the workout because your body temperature is elevated, but within a few hours when you have cooled down, you will be plenty hungry. The more you exercise, the more you will want to eat—be sure to make the time to do so.

6. *Be patient.* If you are in high school or college and don't easily bulk up this year, you may do so more easily as you get

older. Know that you can be a strong rider by being well-fueled and well-trained. Your skinny legs may hurt your self-esteem more than your athletic ability.

● SUMMARY—

- You can change your physique to a certain extent, but first, have a clear picture of your genetic blueprint and a realistic goal. You may be genetically predisposed to be thin—a "hard gainer."
- Just like losing weight, gaining weight takes time, patience, and perseverance.
- The bottom line for gaining weight is to consume more calories than you expend.
- To gain one-half to one pound per week, consume an additional 500 to 1000 calories a day.
- Weight-gain powders are not necessary; you can gain weight healthfully and easily with ordinary supermarket foods.
- Extra exercise, not extra protein, builds bigger muscles.
- Remember these six rules for successful weight gain:
  1. Eat consistently.
  2. Eat larger portions.
  3. Select higher-calorie foods, but not higher-fat foods.
  4. Drink extra juice and low-fat milk.
  5. Do strength training.
  6. Be patient.

CHAPTER 16

In Pursuit of Thinness

ACTIVE PEOPLE OF ALL AGES AND ABILITIES APPRECIATE THE FITNESS, fun, and physical benefits that come with bicycling. Most cyclists have hearty, healthy appetites that support their exercise programs. Good nutrition helps them to:

- attain their goals of racing better, completing a tour, or enjoying a century ride,
- maintain energy to handle their fast-paced lifestyles,
- reduce their risk of injuries, and
- for women, ensure having regular menstrual periods.

But for some cyclists, eating presents challenges. Due to the prevailing myths that thinness contributes to both better performance and happiness, some cyclists consider food to be a fattening enemy rather than a friendly fuel. With the fear that eating meals will make them heavy and slow, they deny themselves permission to eat adequately. Appropriate meals are placed on hold until they lose those final few pounds and feel better about their weight.

Fueled by the "thinner is better" philosophy, cyclists who strive to be abnormally thin commonly pay a high price: eating disorders, poor nutrition, poorly fueled muscles, loss of menses (in women), stress fractures and other injuries, to say nothing of reduced stamina, endurance, and performance. In their over-concern about their weight they forget this formula for success:

appropriate eating + regular exercise = appropriate weight

Chapter 14 offers guidance about how to lose weight and

maintain energy for riding. This chapter provides additional perspective to help resolve the food and weight obsessions of active men and women. The majority of this chapter is targeted to women, because women tend to be very weight-conscious. But if you are a man who struggles with food, the information will help you too.

● **WOMEN AND WEIGHT**—While both male and female cyclists can struggle with weight obsession, women clearly have more issues with food and weight than do men. Let's look at the possible explanations.

1. Women are supposed to have more body fat than men. Plain and simple, nature prescribes to women a certain amount of body fat that is essential for two reasons:
- to protect their ability to create and nourish healthy babies and
- to be a storehouse of calories for pregnancy and breast feeding.

> ❝*When it comes to diet and weight management, I think it's psychologically difficult for female athletes to eat as much as we need to. We've been brain washed to believe eating is bad.* ❞
>
> Tracie Timothy, Salt Lake City, UT

This essential body fat is stored not only in the breasts but also in the hips, abdomen, buttocks, and upper legs, which explains why women have rounder hips and heavier thighs than most men. Women have almost three times as much essential body fat as men: 11 percent to 13 percent of a woman's body weight versus only 3 percent to 5 percent of a man's body weight is essential fat. Women who try to achieve the so-called "cut look" of male athletes create physiological turmoil and commonly pay the price by starving, bingeing, and obsessing about food in order to reach their desired image.

2. Women commonly target an unnatural weight. Women who try to get below their natural weight are the ones most likely to struggle with food and fight the battle with the bulge. Given that even some of those very lean and fast, front-of-the-pack women riders wish they could be lighter, it is not surprising that eating disorders abound. The majority of men, in comparison, seem to be more at peace with their natural weight and, consequently, at peace with food.

3. Women hold distorted body images. The Madison Avenue image that adorns every storefront and magazine ad leads us to believe that nature makes all women universally lean. Any aberration is thought to be a result of gluttony and lack of willpower. Wrong!

Nature makes us in different sizes and shapes, like it or not. If the cyclists who are discontent with their weight could only learn to accept and love their bodies, eating disorders would be rare. Take the story of a food-obsessed female cyclist. At 5-feet, 7-inches tall and 120 pounds (170 centimeters and 55 kilograms), she would lament, "I really wish I could weigh 110 pounds (50 kilograms)." A normal, healthy weight for a woman of her height is 135 pounds (61 kilograms)! She was unable to see that she was already very lean. She was training harder and harder to burn calories and lose body fat. Her training contrasted with that of other cyclists, commonly men, who train primarily to enhance performance, not to reshape their bodies.

● **SLOW METABOLISM WOES**—Frustration with inability to lose weight is common among people who claim they have a slow metabolism and eat less than they "deserve," given their rigorous daily exercise regimen. Perhaps you have heard your buddies express complaints similar to the following:
- I eat less than my friends but I still don't lose weight. There must be something wrong with my metabolism.
- I maintain weight on only 1,000 calories per day. I want to lose a few pounds, but I can't imagine eating any less.
- I ride every day and eat only one meal a day. I can't understand why I don't lose weight.

Is it true that some athletes are energy-efficient? Do they efficiently utilize every calorie they eat so they are able to maintain weight on fewer calories than their counterparts who more unproductively burn them off?

According to Dr. Jack Wilmore, exercise physiologist at the University of Texas at Austin, the energy-efficient athlete does not exist. His research suggests that metabolic rate is closely tied to muscle mass. Dieters who overly restrict calories end up burning muscle tissue for energy and tend to have less muscle mass. Consequently, they require fewer calories. This is particularly true with women who constantly restrict their intake. Plain and simple, athletes who have well-developed muscles require more calories than those who have less muscle.

Other researchers believe that a slower metabolism may be nature's way to conserve calories when too few calories are being eaten. For instance, people who perceive themselves as being energy-efficient commonly complain about being cold all the time, feeling lethargic, and (in women) lacking regular menstrual cycles. These symptoms suggest that their diet is too meager to support normal body functions.

Your solution to the slow metabolism woes comes in finding the right amount of calories and nutrients to support a healthy weight for your body.

● **WOMEN AND AMENORRHEA**—If you are a cyclist or triathlete who previously had regular menstrual periods but have stopped menstruating, you are experiencing amenorrhea.

You may think your period stopped because you are too thin or are exercising too much, but that is not the case. There are plenty of very thin cyclists and elite athletes who do have regular menstrual periods, and studies have shown no body fat differences between athletes who regularly menstruate and those who don't (Sanborn et al. 2000).

Research suggests that amenorrhea is actually a nutritional problem and may be due to eating too little (Loucks 2001). Athletes with amenorrhea often struggle to maintain an

> ## ● RISK FACTORS FOR AMENORRHEA
>
> You are more likely to become amenorrheic if you have any of the following:
> - Restrictive diet
> - Rapid weight loss
> - Low body weight
> - Low percent body fat
> - Rigorous exercise program
> - Irregular menstrual periods even before you started to train hard
> - Significant emotional stress

unhealthy low weight, resulting in inadequate nutrition and
consequently, loss of menses. Indeed, athletic amenorrhea is
sometimes a red flag for an eating disorder. If you feel you
struggle harder than your counterparts to maintain your
desired leanness, realize that you may be eating inadequately
and putting yourself at risk for amenorrhea and all of its associated health problems. If you have stopped having regular
menstrual periods, be sure to consult with your gynecologist
for professional guidance.

● **HEALTH RISKS OF AMENORRHEA**—Although you may deem
amenorrhea a desirable side effect of exercise because you no
longer have to deal with the hassles and possible discomfort of
monthly menstrual periods, amenorrhea can lead to undesir-
able problems that can interfere with your health and ability to
perform at your best. These problems include:
- Almost a three times higher incidence of stress fractures
- Premature osteoporosis (weakening of the bones) that can
  effect your bone health in the not-too-distant future
- Possible higher risk of heart disease
- Inability to conceive should you want to have a baby

If the amenorrhea is caused by the eating disorder anorexia, it
is a symptom of pain and unhappiness in your life. Note that the
absence of at least three consecutive menstrual cycles is part of the
American Psychiatric Association's definition for anorexia.

Amenorrheic women who resume menses do restore some
of the bone density lost during their months of amenorrhea,
particularly if they are younger than seventeen years. But they
do not restore all of it. Your goal should be to minimize the

damages of amenorrhea by eating appropriately and taking the proper steps to regain your menstrual periods. Remember, food is fuel, healthful and health-giving, not a fattening enemy.

● **RESOLVING AMENORRHEA**—The possible changes required to resume menses include:

- Training 5 percent to 15 percent less, for instance, 50 minutes instead of an hour
- Consuming 10 percent more calories each week until you ingest an appropriate amount given your activity level. For example, if you have been eating 1,500 calories a day, eat 150 more calories per day for a total of 1,650 total calories per day during the first week; eat 150 calories more per day for a total of 1,800 calories per day during the second week; 1,950 calories per day during the third week, and so on.
- Choosing more protein-rich foods, particularly red meat and yogurt
- Gaining a few pounds

Some amenorrheic athletes have resumed menses with just reduced exercise and no weight gain. Those who totally stop training, such as happens at the time of an injury, often resume menses within two months. Others resume menstruating after gaining less than five pounds. And despite what you may think, this small amount of weight gain does not result in your "getting fat" and can be enough to achieve better health.

If you have stopped menstruating and believe that poor eating may be part of the problem, see the helpful tips below. You should also consider getting a nutrition checkup with a registered dietitian who specializes in sports nutrition. *Help for Eating Disorders* on page 162.

● **FINDING PEACE WITH FOOD**—If you are a woman who suffers from nutritional amenorrhea, or a man or woman who struggles with

> **❝ I loved being very light, lean, and unburdened by menstrual periods. That is, until I got a stress fracture, then another one, and then a third one. They took forever to heal. I think my poor diet was the problem. I made an effort to eat more protein, like tuna, cottage cheese, and even lean roast beef. I started to feel stronger and eventually got my period in three months and three pounds. I now feel better knowing that my body is healthier inside and functioning the way it should. ❞**
>
> Marcia Jones, New York City

food and weight obsession, these tips may help you to resolve the problem and find peace with your body and with eating.

1. *Throw away the bathroom scale.* Rather than striving to achieve a certain number on the scale, let your body weigh what it weighs. Focus on how healthy you feel and how well you perform, rather than on the number you weigh. Remember, weight is influenced by genetics and is more than just a matter of willpower or a numbers game.

2. *If you have weight to lose, don't crash-diet.* Instead, moderately cut back on your calorie intake by about 20 percent. Females who go on severe diets commonly lose their menstrual periods, suggesting that amenorrhea may be an adaptation to the calorie deficit produced either by low calorie intake alone or by increased energy expenditure via exercise. As outlined in chapter 14, extreme dieting is an ineffective way to lose weight, and it wreaks havoc on your body, performance, and self-esteem. By following a healthy and moderate reducing program, you will have greater success with long-term weight loss and have enough energy to ride and train hard.

3. *If you are at an appropriate weight, practice eating as you did when you were a child: Eat when you are hungry, stop when you are content.* If you are always hungry and are constantly obsessing about food, you are undoubtedly trying to eat too few calories. Your body is complaining and requesting more food. Remember that you need to eat adequate calories to support your training program. Chapter 13 can help you determine an appropriate caloric intake and eating schedule that may differ from your current routine, particularly if you yo-yo between starving and bingeing.

4. *Eat adequate protein.* Research suggests that amenorrheic athletes tend to eat less protein than their regularly menstruating counterparts. Make sure you consume adequate protein (especially if you are vegetarian (see chapter 5). Vegetarian women who consume adequate protein and calories tend to have regular menstrual periods (Barr 1999). If you skimp on protein foods, such as meats and dairy products, your diet also likely lacks iron and calcium and puts you at risk for anemia and osteoporosis.

If you feel you are struggling too much with food and may have an eating disorder, seek help and information by contacting:

National Eating Disorders Association
603 Stewart St., Suite 803
Seattle, WA 98101
Tel: (206) 382-3587
www.nationaleatingdisorders.org

American Dietetic Association
120 South Riverside Plaza, Suite 2000
Chicago, IL 60606-6995
Tel: (800)-877-1600
www.eatright.org

Something Fishy Website on Eating Disorders
www.something-fishy.org

Gürze Books
P.O. Box 2238
Carlsbad, CA 92018
Tel:(800) 756-7533
www.bulimia.com

If you are worried that your training partner or friend is struggling with food issues, speak up! Anorexia and bulimia are self-destructive eating behaviors that may signal underlying depression and can be life-threatening. Here are some helpful tips:

• Approach the person gently but be persistent. Say that you are worried about his/her health. The individual, too, may be concerned about his/her loss of concentration, light-headedness, or chronic fatigue. These health changes are more likely to be a stepping stone to accepting help, since the person clings to food and exercise for feelings of control and stability.

• Don't discuss weight or eating habits. Address the fundamental problems of life.

• Focus on unhappiness as the reason for seeking help. Point out how anxious, tired, and/or irritable the person has been lately. Emphasize that he or she doesn't have to be that way.

• Post a list of resources with tear-off phone numbers at the bottom where the person will see it (see resources listed above).

• Remember that you are not responsible and can only try to help. Your power comes from using community resources and health professionals, such as a counselor, nutritionist, or eating disorders clinic.

5. Eat at least 20 percent of your calories from fat. Plenty of athletes think that if they eat fat, they will get fat. Amenorrheic athletes commonly avoid meat and other protein-rich foods because they are afraid of eating fat. Although excess calories from fat are easily fattening, some fat (20 percent to 30 percent of total calories) is an appropriate part of a healthy sports diet. For most active people, this translates into 40 to 60 or more grams of fat per day. A little fat in the diet tastes good, gives a feeling of satisfaction, and can help protect health by providing important nutrients. Clearly, this differs from a no-fat diet and allows moderate amounts of lean meats, peanut butter, nuts, olive oil, and other wholesome foods that balance a sports diet.

On the opposite extreme, do not eat too much fat, thinking carbohydrates are fattening and eating fat helps burn fat. Eating too much fat (or protein, for that matter) displaces the carbohydrates you need to fuel your muscles. Refer to chapter 6 for more information on fat and chapter 5 for more on protein.

6. Include small portions of lean red meat two to four times per week. Surveys of runners show that those with amenorrhea tend to eat less red meat and are more likely to follow a vegetarian diet than their regularly menstruating counterparts (Kaiserauer et al. 1989). Among nonrunners, vegetarian women are five times more likely to have menstrual problems than meat eaters (Barr 1999). Some researchers believe a high-fiber vegetarian diet can alter the hormones that affect menses, estrogen in particular.

7. Maintain a calcium-rich diet. Men and women alike should choose a high-calcium diet to help maintain bone density. Your bones benefit from the protective effect of exercise, but exercise does not compensate for lack of calcium in the diet. Target at least three to four eight-ounce (240-milliliter) servings of milk or yogurt, or other calcium-rich foods each day. See chapter 1 for calcium guidelines.

Although you may cringe at the thought of spending so many calories on dairy foods, remember that low-fat milk is a wholesome food that contains many important nutrients and contributes to fat loss, not gain. Research suggests women who consume three or more servings of milk or yogurt per day tend to be leaner than those who do not (Pereira et al. 2002). If you are eating a very high-fiber diet that includes lots of bran cereal, fruits, and vegetables, you may have an even higher need for calcium because the fiber may interfere with calcium absorption.

You should know that calcium is only one of several factors that affects bone density. There is a genetic factor to osteoporosis. If your mother or grandmother had osteoporosis, you are more likely to develop the condition. Being too thin, getting inadequate exercise, and having low levels of estrogen also contribute to your risk for osteoporosis.

● SUMMARY—

- Due to the prevailing myths that thinness contributes to both better performance and happiness, some cyclists consider food to be a fattening enemy rather than a friendly fuel.
- Cyclists who strive to be abnormally thin commonly pay a high price: eating disorders, poor nutrition, poorly fueled muscles, amenorrhea (in women), stress fractures and other injuries, to say nothing of reduced stamina, endurance, and performance.
- Women are supposed to have more body fat than men, yet often they target unnaturally low weights.
- Amenorrheic athletes often strive to maintain an unhealthy low weight and restrict calories. The changes that may be required to resume menses include eating more calories and protein, reducing training, and gaining weight.
- Rather than striving to achieve a certain number on the scale, let your body weigh what it weighs. Focus on how healthy you feel and how well you perform, rather than on the number you weigh.
- Remember, food is fuel and hunger is your body's request for fuel. Eat when you are hungry and stop when you are satisfied. If you are always hungry and are constantly thinking about food, you are undoubtedly trying to eat too few calories.

To find a sports nutritionist:

American Dietetic Association
120 South Riverside Plaza, Suite 2000
Chicago, IL 60606-6995
Tel.: (800) 877-1600
www.eatright.org (click on Find a
Nutrition Professional)

Catalogs for nutrition information

*Nutrition Counseling and Education
Services (NCES)*
1904 East 123rd Street
Olathe, KS 66061
Tel.: (877) 623-7266
www.ncescatalog.com

Eating Disorders Resource Catalog
Gürze Books
P.O. Box 2238
Carlsbad, CA 92018
Tel.: (800) 756-7533
www.bulimia.com

Human Kinetics
P.O. Box 5076
Champaign, IL 61825-5076
Tel.: (800) 747-4457
www.humankinetics.com

Cycling organizations

Adventure Cycling Association
150 East Pine Street
P.O. Box 8308
Missoula, MT 59802
Tel.: (800) 755-2453 (toll-free)
www.adventurecycling.org

Adventure Cycling's mission is to inspire people of all ages to travel by bicycle. They organize tours, run instructional and leadership programs, and provide information and inspiration for cyclists. Their National Bicycle Route Network encompasses more than 33,000 miles of roads perfectly suited for cycling. Their *Adventure Cyclist* magazine is published nine times a year. Check out the Cyclosource Online Store for maps, gear, books and more.

League of American Bicyclists
1612 K Street NW
Suite 800
Washington, DC 20006-2850
Tel.: (202) 822-1333
www.bikeleague.org

Through advocacy and education, LAB works to promote bicycling for fun, fitness, and transportation.

Randonneurs USA
c/o Bill Bryant
226 West Avenue
Santa Cruz, CA 95060
Tel.: (831) 425-2939
www.rusa.org

RUSA provides resources and information for non-competitive, long-distance, unsupported endurance cycling (randonneuring).

UltraMarathon Cycling Association, Inc.
P.O. Box 18028
Boulder, CO 80308-1028
Tel.: (303) 545-9566
www.ultracycling.com

UMCA promotes the sport of long-distance bicycling. They sanction and promote ultracycling events, including the Race Across AMerica (RAAM). UltraCycling magazine provides information and support for the endurance cyclist. The UltraMarathon Cycling Association is open to anyone interested in long distance cycling, from century rides to RAAM.

USA Cycling
One Olympic Plaza
Colorado Springs, CO 80909
Tel.: (719) 866-4581
www.usacycling.org

USA Cycling is a family of bicycle racing organizations: National Off-Road Bicycle Association; United States Cycling Federation; United States Professional Racing Organization; and National Collegiate Cycling Association. USA Cycling promotes and governs the sport of bicycling racing and assists with athlete development.

Recommended reading

Benardot, D. 2002. *Nutrition for Serious Athletes*. Champaign, IL: Human Kinetics

Burke, E. 2002. *Serious Cycling*. Champaign, IL: Human Kinetics

Bittman, M. 1998. *How to Cook Everything: Simple Recipes for Great Food*. New York: Wiley Publishing, Inc.

Clark, N. 2003. *Nancy Clark's Sports Nutrition Guidebook, Third Edition.* Champaign, IL: Human Kinetics

Dorfman, L. 2000. *The Vegetarian Sports Nutrition Guide: Peak Performance for Everyone from Beginners to Gold Medalists.* New York: John Wiley & Sons, Inc.

Doughty, S. 2001. *The Long Distance Cyclists' Handbook.* Guilford, CT: The Globe Pequot Press

Duyff, R. 2002. *The American Dietetic Association Complete Food and Nutrition Guide.* Hoboken, NJ: John Wiley & Sons, Inc.

Fragakis, A. 2003. *The Health Professional's Guide to Popular Dietary Supplements.* Chicago: American Dietetic Association

Friel, J. 1998. *Cycling Past 50 for Fitness and Performance Through the Years.* Champaign, IL: Human Kinetics

Girard Eberle, S. 2000. *Endurance Sports Nutrition.* Champaign, IL: Human Kinetics

Jeukendrup, A., ed. 2002. *High-Performance Cycling.* Champaign, IL: Human Kinetics

Lovett, R. 2001. *The Essential Touring Cyclist: A Complete Course for the Bicycle Traveler.* Camden, ME: Ragged Mountain Press

Masterson, P. 2004. *Bicycling Bliss: Riding to Improve Your Wellness.* Golden, CO: Self Propulsion, Inc.

Rosenbloom, C., ed. 2000. *Sports Nutrition: A Guide for the Professional Working with Active People.* Chicago: American Dietetics Association

Newsletters

Tufts University Health & Nutrition Letter
P.O. Box 420235
Palm Coast, FL 32142-0235
www.healthletter.tufts.edu

University of California Berkeley Wellness Letter
P.O. Box 420148
Palm Coast, FL 32142
www.berkeleywellness.com

Online information

Dietary Analysis:

www.usda.gov/cnpp
Information and interactive tool for comparing your diet to the food

Dietary Supplements:

www.consumerlab.com
Research results of independent testing on nutritional supplements

www.nccam.nih.gov
http://dietary-supplements.info.nih.gov
Scientific information, alerts, and advisories about supplements, herbs, and alternative medicine

Eating Disorders:

www.NationalEatingDisorders.org
www.something-fishy.org

Health, Nutrition, and Healthful Eating:

www.healthfactsandfears.com
Answers to popular nutrition and health questions

www.americanheart.org
Information about a heart-healthy lifestyle

www.mayoclinic.com
Information on nutrition, fitness, and sports nutrition and recipes

www.nlm.nih.gov
Limited access to the latest research in nutrition, medical, and scientific journals

www.navigator.tufts.edu/
Tufts University's rating guide to nutrition websites and books

Sports and Sports Nutrition:

www.ais.org.au/nutrition
www.gssiweb.com
www.sportsci.org
Comprehensive information on physical fitness and nutrition

Vegetarianism:

www.vrg.org
Nonprofit group dedicated to educating the public on vegetarianism

Weight Loss:

www.eatright.org
Use the referral network to find a local sports dietitian who can design a personalized plan to help you lose weight and maintain energy for exercise.

SELECTED REFERENCES

Ainsworth, B., W. Haskell, M. Whitt, M. Irwin, et al. 2000. Compendium of Physical Activities: An update of activity codes and MET intensities. *Med Sci Sports Exerc* 32 (suppl):S498-S516.

American College of Sports Medicine, American Dietetic Association, and Dietitians of Canada. 2000. Joint Position Statement: Nutrition and Athletic Performance. *Med Sci Sports Exerc* 32 (12):2130-2145.

Armstrong, L. 2002. Caffeine, body fluid-electrolyte balance, and exercise performance. *Int J Sports Nutr and Exerc Metab* 12:189-206.

Atkinson, G., R. Davison, A. Jeukendrup, and L. Passfield. 2003. Science and cycling: current knowledge and future directions for research. *J Sports Sci* 21 (9):767-787.

Bahrke, M. and W. Morgan. 2000. Evaluation of the ergogenic properties of ginseng: an update. *Sports Med* 29:113-133.

Barr, S. 1999. Vegetarianism and menstrual cycle disturbances: Is there an association? *Am J Clin Nutr* 70 (suppl): 549S-554S.

Bouchard, C. 1991. Heredity and the path to overweight and obesity. *Med Sci Sports Exerc* 23 (3):285-291.

Burke, L., B. Kiens, J. Ivy. 2004. Carbohydrates and fat for training and recovery. *J Sports Sci* 22 (1):15-30.

Burke, L., G. Collier, E. Broad, et al. 2003. Effect of alcohol intake on muscle glycogen storage after prolonged exercise. *J Appl Physiol* 95 (3):983-990.

Casa, D., L. Armstrong, S. Montain, et al. 2000. National Athletic Trainers Association position statement: Fluid replacement for athletes. *J Athletic Training* 35 (2):212-224.

Davis, J. 1995. Carbohydrates, branched-chain amino acids and endurance: the central fatigue hypothesis. *Int J Sport Nutr* 5:S29-S38.

Dawson, D., et al. 2002. Effect of C and E supplementation on biochemical and ultra-structural indices of muscle damage after a 21 km run. *Int J Sports Med* 23 (1):10-15.

Engels, H-J. and J. Wirth. 1997. No ergogenic effects of ginseng (Panax Ginseng CA Meyer) during graded maximal aerobic exercise. *J Am Dietet Assoc* 97:1110-1115.

Flakoll, P., et al. 2004. Post-exercise protein supplementation improves health and muscle soreness during basic military training in marine recruits. *J Appl Physiol* 96:951-956.

Foster, G., T. Wadden, I. Feurer, et al. 1990. Controlled trial of the metabolic effects of a very-low-calorie diet: short and long term effects. *Am J Clin Nutr* 51:167-172.

Foster-Powel, K., S. Holt, and J. Brand-Miller. 2002. International table of glycemic index and glycemic load values. *Am J Clin Nutr* 76 (1):5-56.

Fragakis, A. 2003. The Health Professionalís Guide to Popular Dietary Supplements. Chicago, IL: *American Dietetic Association*, pp. 45-50.

Godard, M., D. Williamson, et al. 2002. Oral amino-acid provision does not affect muscle strength or size gains in older men. *Med Sci Sports Exerc* 34 (7):1126-1131.

Gretebeck, R., K. Gretebeck, and T. Tittelbach. 2002. Glycemic index of popular sports drinks and energy foods. *J Am Diet Assoc* 102 (3):415-416.

Hargreaves, M., J. Hawley, and A. Jeukendrup. 2004. Pre-exercise carbohydrate and fat ingestion: effects on metabolism and performance. *J Sports Sci* 22 (1):31-38.

Hawley, J. 2002. Effect of increased fat availability on metabolism and exercise capacity. *Med Sci Sports Exerc* 34 (9):1485-1491.

Ivy, J. 2001. Dietary strategies to promote glycogen synthesis after exercise. *Can J Appl Physiol* 26 (suppl):S236-S245.

Ivy, J., H. Goforth, G. Damon, et al. 2002. Early postexercise muscle glycogen recovery is enhanced with a carbohydrate-protein supplement. *J Appl Physiol* 93 (4):1337-1344.

Ivy, J., A. Katz, C. Cutler, W. Sherman, and E. Coyle. 1988. Muscle glycogen synthesis after exercise: effect of time of carbohydrate ingestion. *J Appl Physiol* 64:1480-1485.

Jentjens, R., L. Van Loon, C. Mann, A. Wagenmakers, and A. Jeukendrup. 2001. Addition of protein and amino acids to carbohydrates does not enhance post-exercise muscle glycogen synthesis. *J Appl Physiol* 91:839-846.

Jeukendrup, A., J. Martin. 2001. Improving cycling performance: how should we spend our time and money. *Sports Med* 31 (7):559-569.

Kaiserauer, S., A. Snyder, M. Sleeper, and J. Zierath. 1989. Nutritional, physiological, and menstrual status of distance runners. *Med Sci Sports Exerc* 21 (2):120-125.

Kilduff, L., P. Vidakovic, G. Cooney, et al. 2002. Effects of creatine on isometric bench-press performance in resistance-trained humans. *Med Sci Sports Exerc* 34 (7):1176-1183.

Kirwan, J., D. Cyr-Campbell, et al. 2001. Effects of moderate and high glycemic index meals on metabolism and exercise performance. *Metabolism* 50 (7):849-855.

Koopman R., et al. 2004. Combined ingestion of protein and carbohydrate improves protein balance during ultra-endurance exercise. *Am J Physiol* 287 (4):E712-720.

Levine, J., S. Schleusner, and M. Jensen. 2000. Energy expenditure of nonexercise activity. *Am J Clin Nutr* 72 (6):1451-1454.

Loucks, A. 2001. Physical health of the female athlete: Observations, effects, and causes of reproductive disorders. *Can J Appl Physiol* 26 (suppl):S176-185.

Magal, M., et al. 2003. Comparison of glycerol and water hydration regimens on tennis-related performance. *Med Sci Sports Exerc* 35 (1):150-156.

McManus, K., L. Antinoro, and F. Sacks. 2001. A randomized controlled trial of a moderate-fat, low-energy diet compared with a low-fat, low-energy diet for weight loss in overweight adults. *Int J Obes Metab Disord* 25 (10):1503-1511.

Montner, P., D. Stark, M. Riedesel, et al. 1996. Pre-exercise glycerol hydration improves cycling endurance time. *Int J Sports Med* 17:27-33.

Nieman, D., et al. 2002. Influence of vitamin C supplementation on oxidative and immune changes after an ultramarathon. *J Appl Physiol* 92 (5):1070-1077.

Pereira, M., D. Jacobs, L. Van Horn, et al. 2002. Dairy consumption, obesity and the insulin resistance syndrome in young adults. *JAMA* 287 (16):2081-2089.

Sanborn, C. et al. 2000. Disordered eating and the female athlete triad. *Clin Sports Med* 19 (2):199-213.

Schabort, E., A. Bosch, et al. 1999. The effect of a preexercise meal on time to fatigue during prolonged cycling exercise. *Med Sci Sports Exerc* 31 (3):464-471.

Schwenk, T. and C. Costley. 2002. When food becomes a drug: nonanabolic nutritional supplement use in athletes. *Am J Sports Med* 30:907-916.

Sherman, W., G. Brodowicz, D. Wright, et al. 1989. Effects of 4 h preexercise carbohydrate feedings on cycling performance. *Med Sci Sports Exerc* 21 (5):598-604.

Terjung, R., et al. 2000. American College of Sports Medicine Roundtable. The physiological and health effects of oral creatine supplements. *Med Sci Sports Exerc* 32 (3):706-717.

Wagner, D.R. 1999. Hyperhydrating with glycerol: implications for athletic performance. *J Am Diet Assoc* 99:207-212.

Webster J., T. Scheett, M. Doyle, et al. 1997. The effect of a thiamin derivative on exercise performance. *Eur J Appl Physiol* 75:520-524.

Wee, S., C. Williams, S. Gray, and J. Horabin. 1999. Influence of low and high glycemic index meals on endurance running capacity. *Med Sci Sports Exerc* 31 (3):393-399.

Zachweija, J. 2002. *Protein: Power or puffery?* [Online]. Gatorade Sports Science Institute-Sports Science Center. Available: http://www.gssiweb.com

Sweat rate, 69
Sweet potatoes. *See* Potatoes and
   sweet potatoes
Sweets. *See* Snack foods; Sugar
Table sugar. *See* Sugar
Taste fatigue, on long rides, 98
Thirst, 70, 92, 102
Tofu (table), 54, 65
Tolerating food, 86-90, 96
   See also Gastrointestinal problems;
      Pre-ride food
Tomato sauce, variations to, 119
Training:
   carbohydrate-loading during, 118
   effect on glycogen stores, 117, 120
   experimenting during, 118, 125
   impact on GI problems, 120
   tapering, 120
Traveling, 118, 126-130
Turkey (table), 112
Underweight. *See* Diet, for weight gain
Urine and urination, 70, 84, 102
   See also Hydration; Fluid
U.S. Department of Agriculture (USDA)
   food pyramid.
   See Food guide pyramid
U.S. Food and Drug Administration (FDA),
   39, 43
V-8 juice (table), 71, 109, 112, 113
Variety in diet, 1
   See also Balanced diet; Diet
Vegetables:
   calcium in (table), 10
   cooking, 9
   in dining-out meals, 9
   as iron source (table), 58
   eating more, 8, 9, 30 (table)
   nutritional value of (table), 3, 30, 46,
      64, 65
   servings sizes of, 6
   See also names of specific vegetables
Vegetarian diet. *See* Diet, vegetarian
Vitamin A, 3, 30, 46, 36
Vitamin B-complex, 39, 41, 43, 44
Vitamin C, 36, 44, 58
   sources of (table), 3, 30 38, 46
Vitamin D, 40
Vitamin E, 44, 46 (table)

Vitamin supplements. *See* Supplements,
   of vitamins and minerals
Vitamins:
   dietary sources of (table), 44
   fat soluble, 62
   to enhance health or performance
      42, 44
   as fundamental nutrients, 39
   requirement for, 41
Water, as important nutrient, 68
   See also Fluids
Weight (body weight), target, 141 (table),
   148, 151, 155, 156
Weight-gain diet, 152-154
Weight lifting, for muscle mass, 153
Weight-reduction:
   break from, 147
   counting calories for, 131, 133
   during recovery, 112, 113
   keys for successful, 142-149
   See also Appetite; Calories;
      Food cravings; Hunger
Wheat germ (table), 46, 59
Whole-grains, 5, 16
Wholesome foods, 5, 40
Women, and weight, 149, 156, 157
Yogurt (table), 7, 10, 71, 98, 109, 113
Zinc:
   deficiency of, 52
   sources of, 36, 59

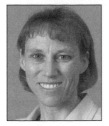

Nancy Clark, MS, RD, an internationally known sports nutritionist, counsels both competitive athletes and casual exercisers in the Boston area. She is consultant to the Boston Red Sox and Boston College's atheletes.

Clark completed her undergraduate degree in nutrition from Simmons College in Boston, her dietetic internship at Massachusetts General Hospital, and her graduate degree in nutrition with a focus on exercise physiology from Boston University. She is a Fellow of the American Dietetic Association and the American College of Sports Medicine.

She is author of the best-seller *Nancy Clark's Sports Nutrition Guidebook, Third Edition*, and *Food Guide for Marathoners: Tips for Everyday Champions*. A regular contributor for *Adventure Cyclist* magazine, Clark also writes a monthly nutrition column called "The Athletes' Kitchen," which appears regularly in over 100 sports and health publications.

A regular bike commuter for over 30 years, Clark has bicycled across America as a tour leader for Adventure Cycling Association, lead several other bike tours, and, as a runner, completed several marathons. She lives in the Boston area with her husband and two children.

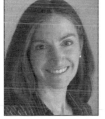

Jenny Hegmann, MS, RD, is a registered dietitian specializing in sports nutrition, wellness, and weight management. She presents nutrition seminars for the public, athletes, and professionals and writes for magazines, newsletters, and medical and fitness websites.

Hegmann completed her undergraduate degree in dietetics from Idaho State University, her dietetic internship at Massachusetts General Hospital, and her graduate degree in human nutrition and metabolism from Boston University. She is a member of the American Dietetic Association and its affiliate, Sports, Cardiovascular, and Wellness Nutritionists.

A serious cyclist for over 20 years, Hegmann has participated in races, randonnées, century rides, triathlons, and weekend tours. She is a member of the Northeast Bicycle Club and faithfully bike commutes from her home in Reading, Mass., to her office in Boston. Hegmann is equally passionate about food and cooking and when not on her bike, can be found in her kitchen dishing up healthy feasts for family and friends.

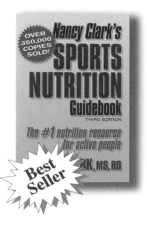

"Nancy Clark's Sports Nutrition Guidebook *is my nutrition bible. It helped me lose weight, improve my eating, boost my energy, and feel stronger."*

If you like *The Cyclist's Food Guide*, you'll also like *Nancy Clark's Sports Nutrition Guidebook, Third Edition*. With more than 350,000 copies in print, this comprehensive resource is divided into four sections:
• daily eating on the run
• sports nutrition for both casual and competitive athletes
• weight management issues and eating disorders
• quick and easy recipes that support healthful eating.

"*Clark's CD on* Dieting Tips for Active People *is actually helpful. I've lost three pounds already and feel more at peace with food."*

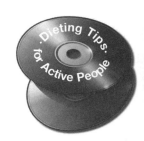

Clark's 40 minute CD can help you have energy to enjoy exercising even when you are losing body fat.

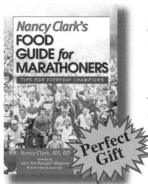

***If your running friends are struggling with low energy, give them* Nancy Clark's Food Guide for Marathoners!**

This easy-reader is perfect for marathoners who want help completing 26.2 miles— as well as the marathon called life.

ORDER FORM: ▬ ▬ ▬ ▬ ▬ ▬ ▬ ▬ ▬ ▬ ▬ ▬ ▬ ▬ ▬

☐ Sports Nutrition Guidebook, $19
☐ Food Guide for Marathoners, $15
☐ Weight loss CD, $10
Postage + $5, $2 every additional item; Mass. residents add 5% sales tax.

Name: _____
Address: _____
City, State, Zip: _____
Phone: _____
email: _____

To order online: www.nancyclarkrd.com

Send check to:
Sports Nutrition Publishing
PO Box 650124
West Newton, MA 02465
Phone: 617-795-0823; Fax: 617-795-1876

Charge to: ☐ Visa ☐ Mastercard

Card number: _____
Exp. Date: _____
Signature: _____

☐ *I'd like more information about Clark's nutrition education materials: handouts and powerpoint presentations on sports nutrition and weight management*